Virtual Medical Office

for

Adams: Kinn's The Administrative Medical Assistant, 8th Edition

Virtual Medical Office

for

Adams: Kinn's The Administrative Medical Assistant, 8th Edition

Study Guide prepared by

Tracie Fuqua, BS, CMA (AAMA)
Program Director
Medical Assistant Program
Wallace State Community College
Hanceville, Alabama

Textbook by

Alexandra Patricia Adams, MA, BA, RMA, CMA (AAMA)

Former Health Information Specialist
Program Director and
Administrative Medical Assisting Instructor
Ultrasound Diagnostic School
(now Sanford-Brown College)

Professional Writer
Grand Prairie, Texas

Software developed by

Wolfsong Informatics, LLC
Tucson, Arizona

ELSEVIER
SAUNDERS

ELSEVIER
SAUNDERS

3251 Riverport Lane
Maryland Heights, Missouri 63043

VIRTUAL MEDICAL OFFICE FOR
ADAMS: KINN'S THE ADMINISTRATIVE MEDICAL ASSISTANT
EIGHTH EDITION

Copyright © 2014, 2011, 2007 by Saunders, an imprint of Elsevier Inc.

ISBN: 978-0-323-22100-9

Notice

Knowledge and best practice in this field are constantly changing. As new research and experience broaden our knowledge, changes in practice, treatment and drug therapy may become necessary or appropriate. Readers are advised to check the most current information provided (i) on procedures featured or (ii) by the manufacturer of each product to be administered, to verify the recommended dose or formula, the method and duration of administration, and contraindications. It is the responsibility of the practitioner, relying on their own experience and knowledge of the patient, to make diagnoses, to determine dosages and the best treatment for each individual patient, and to take all appropriate safety precautions. To the fullest extent of the law, neither the Publisher nor the Authors assumes any liability for any injury and/or damage to persons or property arising out or related to any use of the material contained in this book.

ISBN: 978-0-323-22100-9

Executive Content Strategist: Jennifer Janson
Content Development Strategist: Karen Baer
Publishing Services Manager: Debbie Vogel
Project Manager: Pat Costigan

Printed in the United States of America

Last digit is the print number: 9   8   7   6   5   4   3   2

Table of Contents

GETTING STARTED

The product you have purchased is part of the Evolve Learning System. Please read the following information thoroughly to get started.

■ HOW TO ACCESS YOUR VMO RESOURCES ON EVOLVE

There are two ways to access your VMO Resources on Evolve:

1. If your instructor has enrolled you in your VMO Evolve Resources, you will receive an email with your registration details.

2. If your instructor has asked you to self-enroll in your VMO Evolve Resources, he or she will provide you with your Course ID (for example, 1479_jdoe73_0001). You will then need to follow the instructions at https://evolve.elsevier.com/cs/studentEnroll.html.

■ HOW TO ACCESS THE ONLINE VIRTUAL MEDICAL OFFICE

The Virtual Medical Office simulation is available through the Evolve VMO Resources. There is no software to download or install: the Virtual Medical Office simulation runs within your Internet browser, directly linked from the Evolve site.

■ HOW TO ACCESS THE WORKBOOK

There are two ways to access the workbook portion of *Virtual Medical Office:*

1. Print workbook
2. An electronic version of the workbook, available within the VMO Evolve Resources

■ TECHNICAL SUPPORT

Technical support for *Virtual Medical Office* is available by visiting the Technical Support Center at http://evolvesupport.elsevier.com or by calling 1-800-222-9570 inside the United States and Canada.

1

GETTING SET UP

■ **TECHNICAL REQUIREMENTS**

To use an Evolve Online Product, you will need access to a computer that is connected to the Internet and equipped with web browser software that supports frames. For optimal performance, it is recommended that you have speakers and use a high-speed Internet connection. Dial-up modems are not recommended for *Virtual Medical Office*.

WINDOWS®

Windows PC
Windows XP, Windows Vista™
Pentium® processor (or equivalent) @ 1 GHz (Recommend 2 GHz or better)
800 x 600 screen size
Thousands of colors
Soundblaster 16 soundcard compatibility
Stereo speakers or headphones
Internet Explorer (IE) version 6.0 or higher
Mozilla Firefox version 2.0 or higher

MACINTOSH®

Mozilla Firefox version 2.0 or higher

■ **WEB BROWSERS**

Supported web browsers include Microsoft Internet Explorer (IE) version 6.0 or higher and Mozilla Firefox version 2.0 or higher.

■ SCREEN SETTINGS

For best results, your computer monitor resolution should be set at a minimum of 800 x 600. The number of colors displayed should be set to "thousands or higher" (High Color or 16 bit) or "millions of colors" (True Color or 24 bit).

WINDOWS

1. From the **Start** menu, select **Settings**, then **Control Panel**.
2. Double-click on the **Display** icon.
3. Click on the **Settings** tab.
4. Under **Screen resolution** use the slider bar to select **800 x 600 pixels**.
5. Access the **Colors** drop-down menu by clicking on the down arrow.
6. Select **High Color (16 bit)** or **True Color (24 bit)**.
7. Click on **Apply**, then **OK**.
8. You may be asked to verify the setting changes. Click **Yes**.
9. You may be asked to restart your computer to accept the changes. Click **Yes**.

MACINTOSH

1. Select the **Monitors** control panel.
2. Select **800 x 600** (or greater) from the **Resolution** area.
3. Select **Thousands** or **Millions** from the **Color Depth** area.

Enable Cookies

Browser	Steps
Internet Explorer (IE) 6.0 or higher	1. Select **Tools → Internet Options**. 2. Select **Privacy** tab. 3. Use the slider (slide down) to **Accept All Cookies**. 4. Click **OK**. -OR- 3. Click the **Advanced** button. 4. Click the check box next to **Override Automatic Cookie Handling**. 5. Click the **Accept** radio buttons under **First-party Cookies** and **Third-party Cookies**. 6. Click **OK**.
Mozilla Firefox 2.0 or higher	1. Select **Tools → Options**. 2. Select the **Privacy** icon. 3. Click to expand Cookies. 4. Select **Allow sites to set cookies**. 5. Click **OK**.

Set Cache to Always Reload a Page

Browser	Steps
Internet Explorer (IE) 6.0 or higher	1. Select **Tools → Internet Options**. 2. Select **General** tab. 3. Go to the **Temporary Internet Files** and click the **Settings** button. 4. Select the radio button for **Every visit to the page** and click **OK** when complete.
Mozilla Firefox 2.0 or higher	1. Select **Tools → Options**. 2. Select the **Privacy** icon. 3. Click to expand Cache. 4. Set the value to "**0**" in the **Use up to: __ MB of disk space for the cache** field. 5. Click **OK**.

Plug-Ins

Adobe Acrobat Reader—With the free Acrobat Reader software, you can view and print Adobe PDF files. Many Evolve products offer student and instructor manuals, checklists, and more in this format!

Download at: http://www.adobe.com

Apple QuickTime—Install this to hear word pronunciations, heart and lung sounds, and many other helpful audio clips within Evolve Online Courses!

Download at: http://www.apple.com

Adobe Flash Player—This player will enhance your viewing of many Evolve web pages, as well as educational short-form to long-form animation within the Evolve Learning System!

Download at: http://www.adobe.com

Adobe Shockwave Player—Shockwave is best for viewing the many interactive learning activities within Evolve Online Courses!

Download at: http://www.adobe.com

Microsoft Word Viewer—With this viewer Microsoft Word users can share documents with those who don't have Word, and users without Word can open and view Word documents. Many Evolve products have testbank, student and instructor manuals, and other documents available for downloading and viewing on your own computer!

Download at: http://www.microsoft.com

Quick Office Tour

Welcome to *Virtual Medical Office*, a virtual office setting in which you can work with multiple patient simulations and also learn to access and evaluate the information resources that are essential for providing high-quality medical assistance.

In the virtual medical office, Mountain View Clinic, you can access the Reception area, Exam Room, Laboratory, Office Manager, and Check Out area, plus a separate room for Billing and Coding.

■ BEFORE YOU START

Make sure you have your textbook nearby when you use *Virtual Medical Office* online. You will want to consult topic areas in your textbook frequently while working online and using this study guide.

■ HOW TO SIGN IN

- After entering the access code included inside this study guide, enter your name on the Medical Assistant identification badge.
- Click on **Start Simulation**.

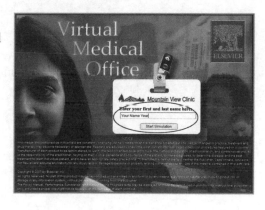

- This takes you to the office map screen. Across the top of this screen is the list of patients available for you to follow throughout their office visit.

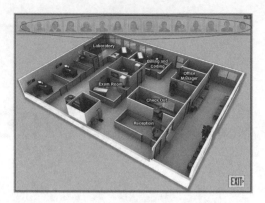

■ PATIENT LIST

1. **Janet Jones (age 50)**—Ms. Jones has sustained an on-the-job injury. She is in pain and impatient. By working with Ms. Jones, students will learn about managing difficult patients, as well as the requirements involved in workers' compensation cases.

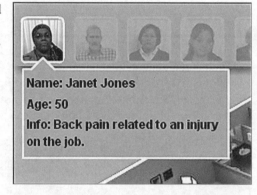

Name: Janet Jones
Age: 50
Info: Back pain related to an injury on the job.

2. **Wilson Metcalf (age 65)**—A Medicare patient, Mr. Metcalf is being seen for multiple symptoms of abdominal pain, nausea, vomiting, and fever. He is seriously ill and might need more specialized care in a hospital setting.

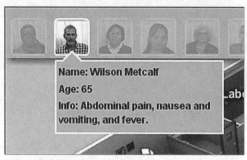

Name: Wilson Metcalf
Age: 65
Info: Abdominal pain, nausea and vomiting, and fever.

3. **Rhea Davison (age 53)**—An established patient with chronic and multiple symptoms, Ms. Davison does not have medical insurance.

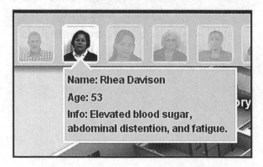

Name: Rhea Davison
Age: 53
Info: Elevated blood sugar, abdominal distention, and fatigue.

4. **Shaunti Begay (age 15)**—A new patient, Shaunti Begay is a minor who has an appointment for a sports physical. Upon arrival, Shaunti and her family learn that Mountain View Clinic does not participate in their health insurance.

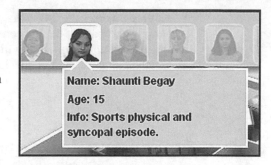
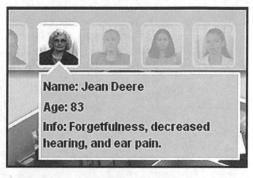

5. **Jean Deere (age 83)**—Accompanied by her son, Ms. Deere is an established Medicare patient being evaluated for memory loss and hearing loss.

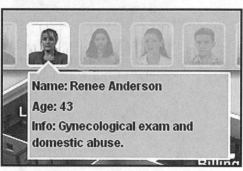

6. **Renee Anderson (age 43)**—Ms. Anderson scheduled her appointment for a routine gynecological examination but exhibits symptoms that suggest she is a victim of domestic violence.

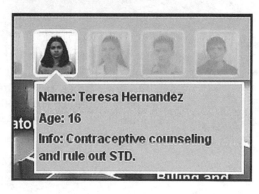

7. **Teresa Hernandez (age 16)**—Teresa is a minor patient who is unaccompanied by a parent for her appointment. She is seeking contraceptive counseling and STD testing.

8. **Louise Parlet (age 24)**—Ms. Parlet is an established patient being seen for a pregnancy test and examination. She will also need to be referred to an OB/GYN specialist.

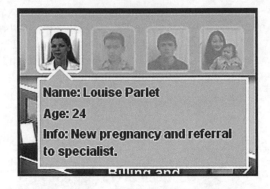

9. **Tristan Tsosie (age 8)**—A minor patient accompanied by his older sister and younger brother, Tristan is having a splint and sutures removed from his injured right arm.

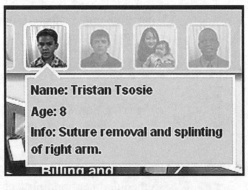

10. **Jose Imero (age 16)**—Jose is a minor patient who is scheduled for an emergency appointment to have the laceration on his foot sutured.

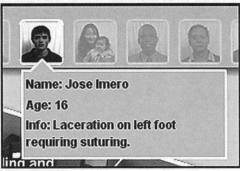

11. **Jade Wong (age 7 months)**—Jade and her parents are new patients to Mountain View Clinic. Jade needs a checkup and updates to her immunizations. Her mother does not speak English.

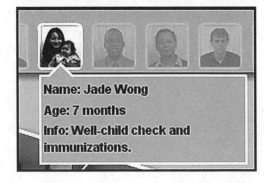

12. **John R. Simmons (age 43)** — Dr. Simmons is a new patient with a history of high blood pressure and recent episodes of blood in his urine.

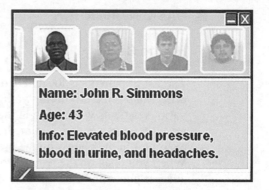

13. **Hu Huang (age 67)** — Mr. Huang developed a severe cough and fever after returning from a recent trip to Asia.

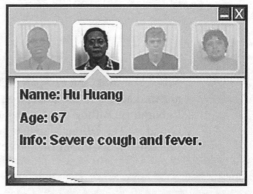

14. **Kevin McKinzie (age 18)** — Mr. McKinzie has made an appointment because of his nausea and vomiting. He is insured through the restaurant where he works.

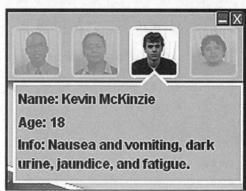

15. **Jesus Santo (age 32)** — Mr. Santo has been brought to the office as a walk-in appointment by his employer for leg pain and a fever. He has no insurance or identification, but his employer has offered to pay for the visit.

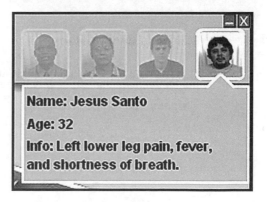

■ BASIC NAVIGATION

How to Select a Patient

The list of patients is located across the top of the office map screen. Pointing your cursor at the various patients will highlight their photo and reveal their name, age, and medical problem (see examples in the photos on the previous pages). When you click on the patient you wish to review, a larger photo and description will appear in the lower left corner of the screen.

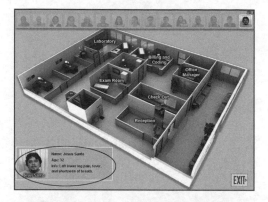

Note: You ***must*** select a patient before you are allowed access to the Reception area, Exam Room, Laboratory, Billing and Coding office, or Check Out area. The Office Manager area is the only room you can enter without first selecting a patient.

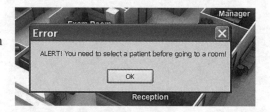

How to Select a Room

After selecting a patient, use your cursor to highlight the room you want to enter. The active room will be shaded blue on the map. Click to enter the room.

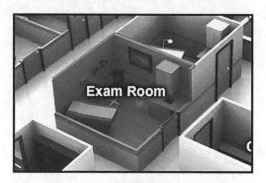

How to Leave a Room

When you are finished working in a room, you can leave by clicking the exit arrow found at the bottom right corner of the screen.

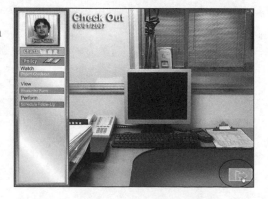

Leaving a room will automatically take you to the Summary Menu.

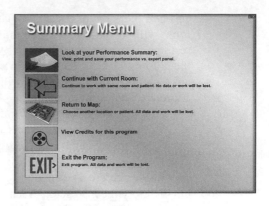

From the Summary Menu, you can choose to:

- **Look at Your Performance Summary**

  In each room there are interactive wizards or tasks that can be completed. The Performance Summary lets you compare your answers with those of the experts.

- **Continue with Current Room**

  This takes you back to the last room in which you worked. This option is not available if you have already reviewed your Performance Summary.

- **Return to Map**

  This reopens the office map for you to select another room and/or another patient.

- **View Credits for This Program**

  This provides a complete listing of software developers, publisher, and authors.

- **Exit the Program**

  This closes the *Virtual Medical Office* software. You will need to sign in again before you can use the program.

HOW TO USE THE PERFORMANCE SUMMARY

If you completed any of the interactive wizards in a room, you can compare your answers with those of the experts by accessing your Performance Summary. The Performance Summary is not a grading tool, although it is valuable for self-assessment and review.

From the Summary Menu, click on **Look at Your Performance Summary**.

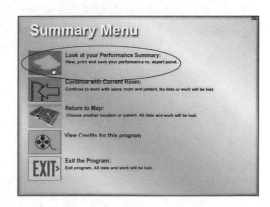

The complete list of tasks associated with the active room will appear with two columns showing the results of your choices. Your answers will appear in the column labeled **Your Performance**, and the answers chosen by the expert will appear in the **Expert's Performance** column. A check mark in the same box in both columns indicates that your answer matched the expert's answer. The Performance Summary can be saved to your computer or disk by clicking on the disk icon at the upper right side of the screen. The saved file can be printed or emailed to your instructor. A hard copy can also be printed without saving by clicking on the printer icon at the upper right corner of the screen.

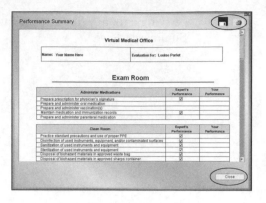

■ ROOM DESCRIPTIONS

Each room can be entered at any time in any order. You can follow a patient's visit from Reception to Check Out, or you can choose to observe each patient at any point in their care. Below is a description of the information and activities that can be found in various rooms.

ALL ROOMS

- In all rooms you can access the patient's medical record and the office Policy Manual.
- In all rooms in which there are interactive tasks to be completed, you can select tasks or features from the menu on the left of the screen, as shown on this sample of the menu in the Reception area.

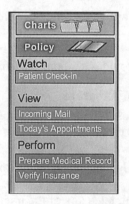

- As an alternative to using the menu, you can click on the corresponding items in the photo of the room. As you move your cursor over each item connected to one of the tasks on the menu, it will highlight and become active.

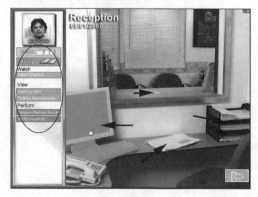

RECEPTION

In the Reception area, you can choose:

- **Charts**—Look at the patient's chart. *Note:* For new patients, there will be no information available in the chart at this time, although you do have the option of assembling a new medical record.
- **Policy**—Open the office Policy Manual and review the established administrative, clinical, and laboratory policies for Mountain View Clinic. Within the Policy Manual you will also find the Coding and Billing Manual.
- **Watch**—Watch a video of the patient's arrival. Each patient is shown checking in at the front desk so that you can observe the procedures typically performed by the receptionist and consider some of the various problems that might arise.
- **Incoming Mail**—Look at the incoming mail for the day. Mountain View Clinic has received a wide range of correspondence that must be read and responded to accordingly.
- **Today's Appointments**—Review the appointment schedule for the day. You can check the schedule to find out what time patients are supposed to arrive, the reason for their visit, and how much time the physician will need for the examination.
- **Prepare Medical Record**—Practice preparing the medical record. This interactive feature allows you to build a medical record for a new patient or update information for an established patient.
- **Verify Insurance**—Verify a patient's insurance. Also interactive, this feature allows you to ask patients about the status of their insurance and to view their insurance cards.

EXAM ROOM

- **Charts** and **Policy**—Access the patient's chart and the office Policy Manual.
- **Watch**—View video clips of different parts of the patient's examination. Observe the actions of the medical assistants in the videos and critique the competencies demonstrated.
- **Exam Notes**—Review the physician's documented findings for the current visit. These notes are added to the full Progress Notes in the patient's chart as the patient continues on to Check Out.
- **Perform**—Perform multiple tasks that are required of a clinical medical assistant, such as preparing the room for the examination, taking vital signs and patient history, and properly positioning the patient for an examination.

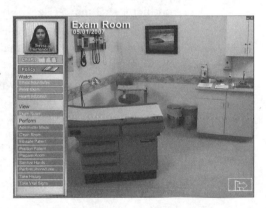

Laboratory

- **Charts** and **Policy**—Access the patient's chart and the office Policy Manual.
- **View: Logs**—View the laboratory's log of specimens sent out for testing. Opportunities to practice filling out laboratory logs are included in the workbook exercises.
- **Perform**—Perform specific tasks as needed in the laboratory, such as collecting and testing specimens. These interactive wizards walk you through the steps for collecting and testing specimens ordered by the physician as part of the patient's examination. The Progress Notes are available throughout so that you can review the physician's directions.

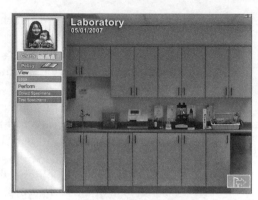

Check Out

- **Charts** and **Policy**—Access the patient's chart and the office Policy Manual.
- **Watch**—Watch a video clip of the patient checking out of the office at the end of the visit. Observe the administrative medical assistants as they schedule follow-up appointments, accept payments, and manage the various duties and problems that may arise.
- **View**—Look at the Encounter Form completed for each patient and verify that the form is filled out correctly and completely.
- **Perform**—Certain patients will require a return visit to the office. Schedule their follow-up appointments as needed. Opportunities to work with the appointment book and additional scheduling tasks are included in the study guide.

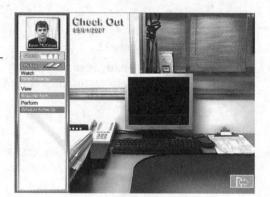

Billing and Coding

- **View: Aging Report**—Review the outstanding balances on various patient accounts and assess when to implement different collection techniques.
- **View: Encounter Form**—Review the patient's Encounter Form and determine whether the proper procedures were followed to ensure accurate billing and coding.
- **View: Fee Schedule**—Review the office's fee schedule to calculate the proper charges for the patient's visit.

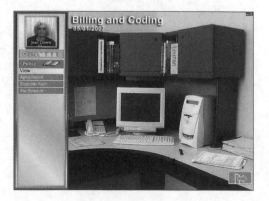

OFFICE MANAGER

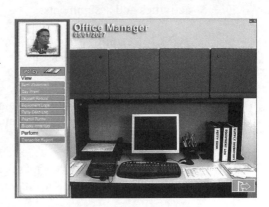

- **Policy**—View the office Policy Manual. Note that patient charts are not available from the manager's office, and there is no need to select a patient to enter the Office Manager area.

- **View**—A variety of financial and administrative documents are available for viewing in the manager's office. Banking deposits and payments can be tracked through these documents, and opportunities to practice managing office finances are included in the study guide.

- **Perform: Transcribe Report**—A recorded medical report is included for transcription practice with full player controls.

■ EMBEDDED ERRORS

The individual lessons and patient scenarios associated with the *Virtual Medical Office* program were designed to stimulate critical thinking and analytical skills and to help develop the competencies on which you will be tested on as part of your course work. Thus deliberate errors have been embedded into each of the 15 patient scenarios and in the Billing and Coding and Office Manager activities. Many of the exercises in the study guide draw attention to these errors so that you can work through how and why a correction needs to be made. Other errors have not been specifically addressed, and you may discover them as you work through the various rooms and tasks. Instructors and students alike are encouraged to use any errors they find to further develop the essential critical thinking and decision-making skills needed for the clinical office.

The following icons are used throughout the study guide to help you quickly identify particular activities and assignments:

 Reading Assignment—tells you which textbook chapter(s) you should read before starting each lesson

 Writing Activity—certain activities focus on written responses such as filling out forms or completing documentation

 Online Activity—marks the beginning of an activity that uses the *Virtual Medical Office* simulation software

 Online Instructions—indicates the steps to follow as you navigate through the software

 Reference—indicates questions and activities that require you to consult your textbook

 Time—indicates the approximate amount of time needed to complete the exercise

Performing Professional Duties

Reading Assignment: Chapter 3—The Medical Assisting Profession
Chapter 4—Professional Behavior in the Workplace
Chapter 5—Interpersonal Skills and Human Behavior

Patient: Rhea Davison

Note: The first exercise does not involve Rhea Davison, but you must choose a patient to access the clinic rooms. We have selected Rhea Davison because she will be your patient later in this lesson.

Learning Objectives:

- Describe the necessary documentation of licensure and accreditation.
- Recognize the need for confidentiality and HIPAA regulations.
- Prepare a travel itinerary for a physician who will be speaking at the national American Association of Medical Assistants (AAMA) conference.
- Locate resources and information for the employer.
- Understand different credentials medical assistants may obtain.

Overview:

In this lesson you will prepare documentation needed for assisting the physician in various areas related to office policies and the physician's professional needs. The ethical and legal aspects of confidentiality are addressed. The Internet will be used to research travel arrangements for a conference one of the physicians needs to attend.

Exercise 1

Online Activity—Maintaining Licensure and Credentials

15 minutes

- Sign in to Mountain View Clinic.
- Select **Rhea Davison** from the patient list.
- Click on **Reception**.
- Under the Watch heading, click on **Patient Check-In** and watch the video.

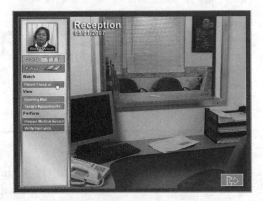

In the video, the medical assistant discusses the CMA (AAMA) credential. However, the RMA is another credential that is recognized on a national level. (*Note:* The CMA credential must now be written as CMA (AAMA) to be distinguished from other CMA credentials that are not Certified Medical Assisting Credentials.)

1. Look up the CMA (AAMA) and RMA credentials and name the organizations that award these credentials. What did you find?

2. Research your state to see if there are any state or regional examinations or credentials awarded by area or region.

3. On arrival this morning, Dr. Meyer states that you need to check on the status of her renewed medical license because it has not arrived. She reminds you that her current license expires on June 1. Go to the Internet and find the name and address of the medical examining board for the state in which you live. Also find the time limit for medical licensure and any necessary components for renewal of the license. Print your findings for your instructor.

4. What are some other credentials medical assistants may obtain?

• Click the **X** on the video screen to close the video.
• Remain in the Reception area with Rhea Davison as your patient to continue to the next exercise.

Exercise 2

 Online Activity—Maintaining Confidentiality and Explaining Office Policy to the Patient

 40 minutes

1. Ms. Davison is an established patient. Did Kristin handle Ms. Davison's late arrival in a professional manner? Explain your answer.

2. Would you have expected Ms. Davison to be upset if her appointment had to be rescheduled?

3. What was your feeling about Kristin and the issue of confidentiality just before the arrival of the office manager?

4. The office manager appeared to be upset with Ms. Davison. However, do you think she was more upset with Ms. Davison or with her employee Kristin? Explain your answer.

5. The office manager explained the need to follow HIPAA policy and the need for confidentiality of medical records. How do you feel about the attitude of the office manager while discussing the matter of confidentiality?

6. Why does the office manager need to explain the HIPAA policy in such a specific manner?

- Click the exit arrow.
- Click **Return to Map**, then click **Yes** at the pop-up menu to return to the office map or click **Exit the Program**.

Exercise 3

Writing Activity—Obtaining Travel Itineraries and Locating Information for the Physician

90 minutes

1. Prepare and provide a travel itinerary for one of the physicians at Mountain View Clinic, following these steps:
   a. Using the Internet as your tool, make travel arrangements for Dr. Meyer to attend the next American Association of Medical Assistants (AAMA) Conference. Dr. Meyer is scheduled to speak on Saturday afternoon at 4 p.m. and would like to arrive at the airport by noon that day. She plans to spend one night and would like a return flight on Sunday arriving no later than 7 p.m.
   b. Decide on the best flight to meet Dr. Meyer's needs from your site (your geographic location) of practice. Record the fare, times of departure and arrival, and any special identification or security requirements.
   c. Make arrangements for Dr. Meyer at the hotel where the conference is being held, showing the room fee including taxes. Make a notation of the check-in time and the check-out time at the hotel.
   d. Finally, arrange for land transportation for Dr. Meyer from the airport to the hotel and back to the airport. Some hotels have a complimentary shuttle or can recommend a shuttle company. You can also check the price of renting a car or the approximate cost for taxi service.

ACP Internal Medicine Meeting   May 5-7, 2016

2. Travel restrictions and requirements change frequently, particularly for travel outside of the United States. Using the Internet as a resource, locate websites that provide updated information on security, restrictions, and requirements for travelers.

3. Dr. Meyer is scheduled to present a speech on sleep apnea at the conference. She asks you to consult the Internet and find five links she can use as information resources as she prepares her speech. What did you find?

(1)

(2)

(3)

(4)

(5)

LESSON 2

Telephone Techniques

Reading Assignment: Chapter 5—Interpersonal Skills and Human Behavior
- The Process of Communication

Chapter 9—Telephone Techniques

Patients: Louise Parlet, Wilson Metcalf

Learning Objectives:

- Describe how nonverbal and verbal communication are apparent when using the telephone.
- Understand the need for ethical and legal behavior on the telephone.
- Identify ways to ensure confidentiality when using the telephone in the medical office.
- Manage telephone calls professionally while handling other administrative duties.

Overview:

In this lesson the legal and ethical issues related to the use of the telephone will be discussed. Issues of confidentiality when using the phone to make arrangements for transfer of a patient to an inpatient facility will also be covered. Proper telephone techniques are important in setting the mood for the entire office. This lesson is designed to provide basic understanding of these techniques.

Exercise 1

Online Activity—Proper Use of the Telephone in the Medical Office

 40 minutes

- Sign in to Mountain View Clinic.
- Select **Louise Parlet** from the patient list.
- Click on **Reception**.
- Under the Watch heading, click on **Patient Check-In** and watch the video.

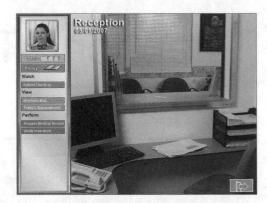

1. As Kristin answers the phone, how does she identify herself? Was her identification a correct procedure? Why or why not?

2. What nonverbal communication does Kristin convey when she answers the phone?

3. Kristin did not close the privacy window while talking on the telephone. Was this a break in confidentiality? Why or why not?

4. When should the privacy window be closed when the medical assistant is on the telephone?

5. Kristin said "Please excuse me" so that she could answer the telephone. When she completed the phone call, she apologized for the interruption. Was this a proper telephone technique? Give a reason for your answer.

6. What was your opinion about the way the sales representative behaved while Ms. Parlet was at the counter?

7. Could Kristin have handled the sales representative's intrusion into their conversation in a more sensitive way from Ms. Parlet's perspective?

8. Assume that Kristin is engaged in a phone call that involves personal information about the medical condition of a patient. How can she determine whether she is communicating with a person to whom she can legally and ethically release the information?

 • Click the **X** on the video screen to close the video.
• Click the exit arrow.
• Click **Return to Map** and select **Yes** at the pop-up menu to return to the office map.
• Select **Wilson Metcalf** from the patient list.
• Click on **Check Out**.
• Under the Watch heading, click on **Patient Check-Out** and watch the video.

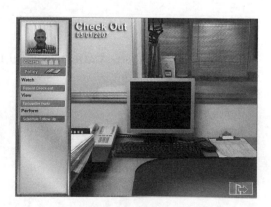

9. How is Mr. Metcalf's confidentiality safeguarded while the medical assistant is on the telephone?

10. How did the medical assistant verify the exact location of the patient transfer so that the orders could be sent as needed?

 • Click the **X** on the video screen to close the video.
- Click on **Charts**.
- Click on the **Patient Medical Information** tab and select **7-Release of Information Authorization**.

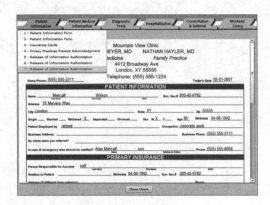

11. Was it permissible for Leah to call Mr. Metcalf's son concerning his transfer to the hospital? Why or why not?

 • Click on the **Patient Medical Information** tab and select **1-Patient Information Form**.

12. What telephone number was given for Mr. Metcalf's son Alan?

13. Would it have been better, in your opinion, to have Mr. Metcalf's son's phone number on the Release of Information Authorization? Why?

 • Click **Close Chart** to return to the Check Out area.
 • Click **Return to Map**, then click **Yes** at the pop-up menu to return to the office map or click **Exit the Program**.

Exercise 2

 Writing Activity

 15 minutes

1. List different acceptable ways to introduce yourself if you were working at Mountain View Clinic, keeping in mind the rules for answering the phone that are discussed in your textbook. Practice each way out loud while holding the telephone. Choose which introduction seems most comfortable to you and be prepared to share your personal preference with your classmates.

2. What do most incoming calls pertain to in the medical office?

3. How far should the medical assistant hold the telephone receiver from his or her mouth when speaking into the handset?

4. List seven vital pieces of information to include on a telephone message.

5. Which types of calls require operator assistance?

6. When possible, why should operator-assisted calls be avoided?

Scheduling and Managing Appointments

Reading Assignment: Chapter 10—Scheduling Appointments

Patient: Janet Jones

Learning Objectives:

- Discuss the rationale for providing space in a day's appointment schedule for emergency appointments.
- Explain the need for a matrix on the appointment schedule.
- Describe the role of the Policy Manual in appointment scheduling.
- Explain the importance of verbal communication concerning appointment delays.
- Apply the skills of scheduling appointments in person and by telephone.
- Apply the skills of maintaining the appointment book.
- Identify office policies concerning rescheduling appointments.
- Apply the skills of rescheduling appointments.

Overview:

In this lesson you will schedule and manage appointments using the policies established for this office. The patient, Janet Jones, is upset because she has not been seen immediately. You will discuss the proper way to deal with such a situation. After today's appointment, Janet Jones will need to come back for a follow-up appointment. You will schedule this appointment for her at the appropriate time and schedule other appointments for established and new patients.

Exercise 1

Online Activity—Using a Specific Daily Appointment Schedule

 25 minutes

- Sign in to Mountain View Clinic
- Select **Janet Jones** from the patient list.
- Click on **Reception**.
- Click on the **Computer**.
- Scroll down the appointment book to see both the morning and afternoon schedules.

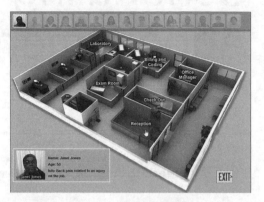

1. According to the appointment schedule, what time is Janet Jones' appointment?

2. If Janet Jones signed in at 1:30 p.m., would she have been on time for her appointment? Explain your answer.

- Click **Finish** to return to the Reception area.
- Under the Watch heading, click on **Patient Check-In** and watch the video.

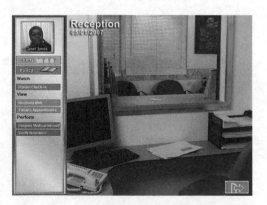

3. Janet Jones is upset when she arrives at the counter. How does Kristin handle the patient in a professional way through verbal and nonverbal communication?

4. Assuming that Ms. Jones checked in at 1:30 p.m., what would have been an appropriate statement for the receptionist to make to the patient as she checked in to prevent her from becoming so upset?

 • Click the **X** on the video screen to close the video.
   • Click on **Policy** to open the office Policy Manual.
   • Type "appointment scheduling" in the search bar and click on the magnifying glass.
   • Read the section of the Policy Manual on scheduling appointments.
   • Keep the Policy Manual open to answer the following questions.

5. What is the length of time needed for an appointment during which a history and physical examination must be completed for a new patient?

6. Why is it necessary to set up a matrix before making appointments?

7. What buffer times are available for emergency appointments, and why is it important to have this time available?

8. According to the office Policy Manual, what would have been appropriate concerning rescheduling Janet Jones' appointment?

9. Why is it important to identify workers' compensation appointments at the time of scheduling rather than at the time of the appointment?

10. Is the patient's time just as valuable as the physician's time? Explain your answer.

→ • Click **Close Manual** to return to the Reception area.
  • Click the exit arrow.
  • Click **Return to Map** and select **Yes** at the pop-up menu to return to the office map.

Exercise 2

Writing Activity—Adding Appointments to a Schedule

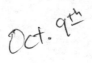

20 minutes

At the end of the day on April 31, a list of patients needing appointments on May 1 was shown to Dr. Hayler and Dr. Meyer. Both physicians stated that because few patients were currently in the hospital, they would be able to see patients in the clinic earlier than usual the next morning. Dr. Hayler and Dr. Meyer will begin seeing patients at 8:15 a.m. The staff has been informed of the early start. The white areas of the appointment book indicate buffer times for adding patients who need to see the doctor today or for those patients with emergent needs. You may choose a patient, go to the Reception desk, open the Policy Manual, and type "appointment scheduling" in the search bar to review the length of time you will need to block off for each appointment.

1. a. Insert the following appointments for Dr. Hayler into the morning schedule on the next page.

   (1) Robert Leuker is a patient who has not been to the clinic in 5 years and wants to be seen for a lump in his arm. He has a past history of cancer and needs to be seen ASAP. He should be seen first in the morning so that he can be referred as necessary. He is insured through BlueCross/BlueShield (BC/BS). His phone number is (555) 555-8890.

   (2) Lindsey Repp needs a follow-up appointment for an earache and recurrent fever. She is insured through Central Health HMO and can be double-booked at the end of the appointment for Louise Parlet. Her telephone number is (555) 555-9004.

   (3) John Price, who needs a follow-up appointment for his blood pressure, has Medicare. His blood pressure was low when he took it yesterday, and he feels dizzy. He simply wants Dr. Hayler to reevaluate his medication. After discussing this with Dr. Hayler, he can be seen just before lunch and will be "worked in" with the other scheduled patients. Mr. Price's phone number is (555) 555-1998.

   b. After completing Dr. Hayler's appointments, add the following appointments for Dr. Meyer in the morning, using the same schedule on the next page.

   (1) Catherine Lake needs a follow-up appointment for pyelonephritis. She forgot to make her follow-up appointment when she was last seen. Ms. Lake is going out of town for 2 weeks and needs to see Dr. Meyer before leaving. Her insurance coverage is through BC/BS. Dr. Meyer will see her at the earliest appointment time. Catherine Lake's phone number is (555) 555-1865.

   (2) Lucille Meryl needs to be seen for a follow-up to a thyroid test. Dr. Meyer wants to see her as a double-booking at the end of the appointment for Rhea Davison. Her insurance is through Drake. Her phone number is (555) 555-3219.

   (3) An established patient, Simon Reed, calls at 11:30 a.m. to tell you that he has some chest pain, and even though he has an appointment for tomorrow, he does not think he should wait. Mr. Reed has experienced a heart attack in the past. When you discuss this with Dr. Meyer, she tells you to phone 911 while keeping the patient on the line. She also says that she will go to the hospital to see Mr. Reed once he is in the emergency room. What notation should you make on the schedule?

Oct. 9th (handwritten)

| | Dr. Hayler | | Dr. Meyer | |
	Name	Insurance	Name	Insurance
8:00 AM	(Hospital rounds) Joe Smitty- Chem 12, CBC Marsha Brady-fasting BS		(Hospital rounds)	
8:15 AM	(Hospital rounds)		(Hospital rounds) Joanne Crosby-PT, PTT	
8:30 AM	Louise Parlet - Est. Pt. New pregnancy/pelvic (555) 555-3214	Teachers'	Rhea Davison - Est. Pt. Elevated blood sugar, abdominal distention, pelvic- (555) 555-5656	None
8:45 AM				
9:00 AM				
9:15 AM				
9:30 AM			Hu Huang - Est. Pt. Severe cough, fever (555) 555-1454	Medicare
9:45 AM	Jade Wong - NP 7 mos. well child checkup/ immunization- (555) 555-3345	Central Health HMO		
10:00 AM			~~Chris O'Neil - back pain~~ (pt. cancelled- resched 5/7) Jesus Santo - NP Leg pain, SOB (walk-in)	None
10:15 AM				
10:30 AM			Jean Deere - Est. Pt. Memory loss, ear pain (555) 555-6361	Medicare
10:45 AM	Tristan Tsosie - Est. Pt. Suture removal (555) 555-1515	BC/BS		
11:00 AM				
11:15 AM			Wilson Metcalf - Est. Pt. N/V, abdominal pain, difficulty urinating- (555) 555-3311	Medicare
11:30 AM	LUNCH			
11:45 AM				
12:00 PM				

2. You must now call John Price to inform him that Dr. Hayler will see him just before lunch. Below, write the information that Mr. Price will need to be told. Why did Dr. Hayler need to be contacted before making the appointment for Mr. Price?

3. You must also call Lucille Meryl to inform her that Dr. Meyer wants to see her about her test results. What information do you need to provide, and how would you answer her if she questions why she needs to be seen so quickly?

Exercise 3

Online Activity—Preparing an Appointment Schedule

30 minutes

- Select **Janet Jones** from the patient list.
- Click on **Check Out**.
- Click on the **Encounter Form** clipboard.

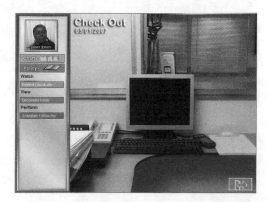

1. What is the date that Janet Jones should return to the clinic for a follow-up appointment?

2. How much time should be allotted to the follow-up appointment for Ms. Jones?

 • Click **Finish** to return to the Check Out area.
• Under the Watch heading, click on **Patient Check-Out** and watch the video.

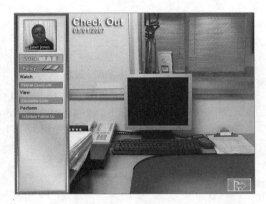

3. At what time of day was Ms. Jones' follow-up appointment made?

 • Click the **X** on the video screen to close the video.
• Click the exit arrow.
• Click **Return to Map** and select **Yes** at the pop-up menu to return to the office map or click **Exit the Program**.

Complete the following activities using the appointment sheets in questions 4 and 5 on the next two pages.

(1) Set up the appointment sheet for the date that Janet Jones is to return for her follow-up visit at the same time the medical assistant in the video scheduled her appointment.

(2) Using the information in the Policy Manual, set up the matrix for that day. (*Note:* If you need to review this, return to the Policy Manual, type "hours of operation" in the search bar, and click once on the magnifying glass.

(3) Add an appointment at 11:00 a.m. for Kay Soto (an established patient) with Dr. Meyer. Ms. Soto has been prescribed a weight loss program and is coming in for a weight check. Her insurance is through Metro HMO. Ms. Soto's phone number is (555) 555-0054.

(4) George Smith, age 15, is to be seen by Dr. Hayler for a football injury the night before. He has State Agricultural Insurance and is an existing patient. George needs to be seen as early as possible so that he can go to school. Mr. Smith's phone number is (555) 555-8778.

(5) Callie Agree, a new patient, is to be seen for a possible sinus infection. She has Medicare and will be accompanied by her daughter. The daughter prefers to see Dr. Meyer in the midmorning so that her mother will have time to dress. Ms. Agree's phone number is (555) 555-3452.

(6) Sophie Coats, age 6 months, is an established patient who will be seen by Dr. Hayler for a well-baby visit. She is due to have immunizations at this visit. Her mother prefers to have an appointment as early in the morning as possible. Sophie is covered by her father's insurance with Banker's Health. Ms. Coats' phone number is (555) 554-0090.

(7) Mamie Mack, age 18, is an established patient who needs a physical examination for college. She prefers to be seen by Dr. Hayler. Either late morning or early afternoon is better for her since she is still in school. She is covered through George Allen Insurance at her mother's place of employment. Ms. Mack's phone number is (555) 554-8745.

(8) Kay Soto calls to cancel her appointment for the day because she has to leave town to take care of her ill mother. She does not want to reschedule at this time.

(9) Dr. Hayler will need to leave at 11:15 a.m. for a dental appointment but will be back in the afternoon by 1:00 p.m. Mark this on the appointment sheet.

(10) Dr. Meyer is scheduled to be off the afternoon of this day. Mark this on the appointment sheet.

4.

/ /2007	Dr. Hayler			Dr. Meyer		
Time	Patient Name		Insurance	Patient Name		Insurance
8:00 AM						
8:15 AM						
8:30 AM						
8:45 AM						
9:00 AM						
9:15 AM						
9:30 AM						
9:45 AM						
10:00 AM						
10:15 AM						
10:30 AM						
10:45 AM						
11:00 AM						
11:15 AM						
11:30 AM						
11:45 AM						
12:00 PM						
12:15 PM						

5.

/ /2007	Dr. Hayler			Dr. Meyer		
Time	Patient Name		Insurance	Patient Name		Insurance
12:30 PM						
12:45 PM						
1:00 PM						
1:15 PM						
1:30 PM						
1:45 PM						
2:00 PM						
2:15 PM						
2:30 PM						
2:45 PM						
3:00 PM						
3:15 PM						
3:30 PM						
3:45 PM						
4:00 PM						
4:15 PM						
4:30 PM						
4:45 PM						
5:00 PM						

6. What is the necessary procedure for canceling Kay Soto's appointment?
   a. Erase the canceled appointment and tell Ms. Soto that there will be a charge because she did not give 24 hours notice.
   b. Cross out the appointment (using the office-preferred writing implement) and record the cancellation in the patient medical record or in the database if using electronic records.
   c. Report the cancellation to Dr. Meyer.
   d. Tell her that she must reschedule this appointment today for continued medical care.

7. Why is it important to document a canceled appointment in the patient's medical record?

8. When is it appropriate to report a canceled appointment to the physician?

Scheduling Admissions and Procedures

Reading Assignment: Chapter 10—Scheduling Appointments
- Scheduling Other Types of Appointments

Chapter 14—The Paper Medical Record
- Releasing Medical Record Information

Patients: Wilson Metcalf, Shaunti Begay

Learning Objectives:

- Recognize the patient information that needs to be sent to a medical facility if your office is making a referral.
- Check the patient's records to verify who is authorized by the patient to receive information regarding the patient.
- Use the Policy Manual to determine the responsibility of the medical assistant in making arrangements for inpatient admissions and referrals to other physicians.
- Explain why it is important to arrange outpatient appointments at a time convenient for the patient.
- Recognize confidentiality issues that must be followed when making arrangements to transfer a patient to a hospital.

Overview:

In this lesson you will make the necessary arrangements for moving Wilson Metcalf from the office to the hospital. You will ensure that his family has been notified of the move. With Shaunti Begay, you will make arrangements for outpatient testing and schedule an office appointment for providing her test results. This patient will also need to see a specialist, so any questions concerning the insurance for these appointments will need to be answered.

Exercise 1

 Online Activity—Scheduling Inpatient Admissions and Procedures

 30 minutes

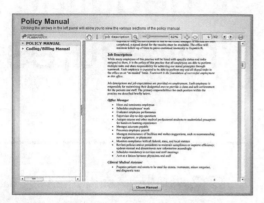

- Sign in to Mountain View Clinic.
- Select **Wilson Metcalf** from the patient list.
- Click on **Check Out**.
- Click on **Policy** to open the office Policy Manual.
- Type "job description" in the search bar and click once on the magnifying glass.
- Read the section of the Policy Manual on the job descriptions for the medical assistants.

1. According to office policy, which medical assistant has the primary duty of making the arrangements for inpatient admissions and for making referrals to other physicians?

→ • Click **Close Manual** to return to the Check Out area.
  • Under the Watch heading, click on **Patient Check-Out** and watch the video. (*Note:* You may have already watched this video in Lesson 2. Review to answer the following question.)

2. Which documents are being copied and sent to the hospital with Mr. Metcalf? Select all that apply.

_____ Medicare card

_____ Private insurance card

_____ Authorization form

_____ Office registration

_____ Physician's orders

- Click on **Charts**.
- Click on the **Patient Information** tab and select **3-Insurance Cards**. Click on **next card** to view the second card.
- Click on the **Patient Information** tab and select **1-Patient Information Form**.
- Click on the **Patient Information** tab and select **6-Release of Information Authorization Form**.
- Note that both the Patient Information Form and the Release of Information Authorization Form are dated 5-1-2007.

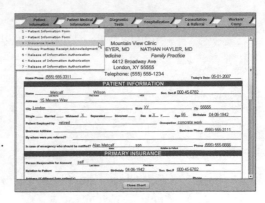

3. Why would it be appropriate to send the office registration and authorization form to the hospital for Wilson Metcalf's admission?

4. Who may receive information concerning Mr. Metcalf's medical condition? Can the entire medical record be released?

5. Did Leah act within the ethical and legal boundaries to release the information she gave to the hospital for Mr. Metcalf? Explain your answer.

6. Why is it important that the window to the waiting room be closed while Leah is making arrangements for Mr. Metcalf to be transferred to the hospital?

→ • Click **Close Chart** to return to the Check Out area.
• Click the exit arrow.
• Click **Return to Map** and select **Yes** at the pop-up menu to return to the office map.

Exercise 2

Online Activity—Scheduling Outpatient Admissions and Procedures

 20 minutes

• Select **Shaunti Begay** from the patient list.
• Click on **Check Out**.
• Click on **Charts**.
• Click on the **Patient Medical Information** tab and select **2-Progress Notes**.

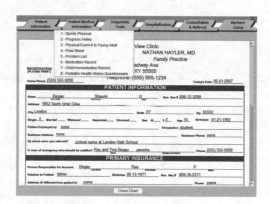

1. What appointments does the check-out medical assistant need to make?

2. Why is it important for Leah to obtain a referral preauthorization, or precertification for the tests to be performed?

3. From the Progress Notes, what patient diagnosis is the physician interested in "ruling out" by this referral?

→ • Click **Close Chart** to return to the Check Out area.
 • Under the Watch heading, click on **Patient Check-Out** and watch the video.

4. Did Leah make sure the referral for outpatient admission and procedures was scheduled at a time convenient for the patient and her family?

Critical Thinking Question

5. Why is it important to check that referrals and appointments to specialists are made at a time that is convenient for the patient?

6. Why is it important to document a canceled appointment in the patient's medical record?

7. Shaunti's father, Mr. Begay, is concerned with the financial aspects of the visit since his insurance is not a provider for this medical office. Leah provided the information about his insurance carrier and the referral. However, she did not provide information that was needed to assist Shaunti in the referral. Can you name two items that were not discussed with or given to Mr. Begay?

8. Refer to the Progress Notes and then look at the referral authorization in Shaunti's chart; compare it with the Progress Notes. Did Leah gain approval for all the tests the doctor wants the patient to have?

9. Mr. Begay was concerned about the amount of the bill for Shaunti. Do you think that Leah was professional in her handling of verbal and nonverbal communication in this interaction? In what way, if any, would you have changed what was said or done? Did Leah act in an ethical manner?

 • Click the **X** on the video screen to close the video.

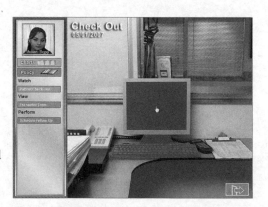

- Click on the **Encounter Form** clipboard.
- Review the information necessary to schedule a follow-up visit.
- Click **Finish** to return to the Check Out area.
- Click on the **Computer**.
- Use the checkboxes to select the actions required to schedule the patient's next visit.
- Click **Finish** to return to the Check Out area.
- Click the exit arrow.
- On the Summary Menu, click on **Look at Your Performance Summary**.
- Scroll down the Performance Summary and compare your answers with those chosen by the experts. The summary can be printed or saved for your instructor.
- Click **Close** to return to the Summary Menu.
- Click **Return to Map**, then click **Yes** at the pop-up menu to return to the office map or click **Exit the Program**.

5

Maintaining a Proper Inventory

○⌒○ **Reading Assignment:** Chapter 12—The Office Environment and Daily Operations
- Supplies and Equipment in the Physician's Office

Patients: None

Learning Objectives:

- Describe the steps necessary for replenishing supplies.
- Discuss how having too many or too few supplies can affect the efficiency of the office.
- Decide which items to reorder and the amount to reorder.
- Explain the necessity of checking equipment for maintenance on a regular basis.
- Discuss the role of the medical assistant in suggesting new equipment for the medical office.
- Describe the proper disposal of controlled substances that are found to be out of date.

Overview:

Ensuring the availability of supplies and equipment when needed is essential to the efficiency of the medical office practice. The proper inventory of supplies and equipment helps to ensure their availability. In some cases, it is more efficient to order supplies in larger quantities. The medical assistant also has the responsibility of making sure that the equipment ordered is the most currently used in the field. Finally, when medications are found to be out of date, proper disposal is necessary. This lesson will focus on supplies and equipment and their importance to office efficiency.

Exercise 1

Online Activity—Deciding When to Replenish Supplies

 30 minutes

- Sign in to Mountain View Clinic.
- Click on **Office Manager**.
- Click on the **Supply Inventory** binder.
- To view the record for each item in the inventory, click on the corresponding tab headings.

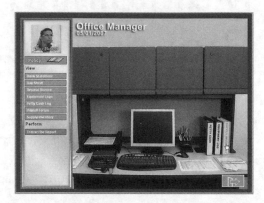

1. What is the reorder point for sutures?

2. Looking at the record from 2006, how many packages of sutures were previously used in May?

➡ • Click on **Gauze** to view the inventory record.

3. What is the reorder point for gauze?

4. Looking at the record from 2006, how many bags of gauze were previously used in May?

5. The inventory for gauze is recorded as bags, but gauze can also be ordered by the case. How many bags are in one case?

6. What is the unit price? Does this represent the price per bag or the price per case?

7. What is the discount offered for ordering four or more cases of gauze?

8. After looking at the inventory supply sheet for gauze, should gauze be reordered? If so, why and how much? If not, why not? If you reorder, what will be the net amount of the purchase?

➤ • Click on the tab heading for **EKG Paper** to view the inventory record.

9. When was the last order placed for EKG paper? How much was ordered?

10. When was this order received?

11. What is the reorder point for EKG paper?

12. How many packs of EKG paper are currently in inventory?

13. Should EKG paper be reordered now? If so, why? If not, why not? If you reorder, what quantity should be reordered?

14. The order for EKG paper is prepaid. What are some possible reasons for setting up a prepaid order for this item? *Use your critical thinking skills while answering this question.*

➤ • Click on **Envelopes** to view the inventory record.

15. How often does the office normally order envelopes?

16. On February 28, 2007, the office ordered four more boxes of envelopes. When did this order arrive?

17. Why is there so much time between when the order is placed and when the order is received?

18. From what you see on the inventory form, do the envelopes need to be reordered? How could the office lower the price of the envelopes? Do you see a problem with the reorder point, and does this need to be changed? If the envelopes should be reordered in bulk, what would be the price?

 • Click on **Paper** to view the inventory record for copier paper.

19. After examining the inventory supply card for copier paper, what is the cost for three cases?

20. What is the cost for ordering five cases?

21. Below, fill out the purchase order for three cases of copier paper. The shipping fee is $6.00 and the sales tax is 6%.

Office Station

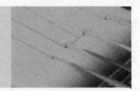

Purchase Order

Bill To:
Mountain View Clinic
4412 Broadway
London, XY 55555

Ship To:
Mountain View Clinic
4412 Broadway
London, XY 55555

Order #:
Date:

Delivery Required By:

Sales Contact	Terms	Tax ID

Item	Quantity	Description	Unit Price	Disc %	Total

Shipping	
Subtotal	
Tax %	
Balance Due	

145 Oceanus Way, St. Pinot, XY 53559
Phone: (123) 456 7890 Fax: (123) 456 7899 CSR@officestation.com

Here is a copy of the supplier's invoice for the copier paper you ordered. Use the information on this invoice to complete question 22 on the next page.

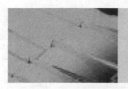 # Office Station

INVOICE #2297

Bill To:
Mountain View Clinic
4412 Broadway
London, XY 55555

Ship To:
Mountain View Clinic
4412 Broadway
London, XY 55555

Order #: **105699**
Date:

Delivery Required By:

Sales Contact	Terms	Tax ID

Item	Quantity	Description	Unit Price	Disc %	Total
CPO-117	3 cases	Copier Paper	$71.27 / 3 cases		$71.27

Shipping	$6.00
Subtotal	$77.27
Tax %	$4.64
Balance Due	$81.91

145 Oceanus Way, St. Pinot, XY 53559
Phone: (123) 456 7890 Fax: (123) 456 7899 CSR@officestation.com

22. Using the information on invoice 2297 from the Office Station (previous page), complete the check below to pay for the delivered supplies.

173980

DATE: _____

TO: _____

FOR: _____

ACCOUNT NO. _____

AMOUNT PAID $ _____

MOUNTAIN VIEW CLINIC
4412 Broadway
London, XY 55555

94-72/1224

173980

Date: _____

Pay to the order of: _____

_____ Dollars $ [   ]

Clarion National Bank
Member FDIC
90 Grape Vine Road
London, XY 55555-0001

_____
Authorized Signature

||⬛ 005503 ||⬛ 4467820ll ||⬛ 678800470

23. How should the ordered supplies be handled when they arrive at the office?

- Click **Finish** to return to the manager's office.
- Click the exit arrow.
- Click **Return to Map** and select **Yes** at the pop-up menu to return to the office map.

Exercise 2

Writing Activity—Properly Disposing Medications

10 minutes

- Sign in to Mountain View Clinic and select any patient from the patient list.
- Click on **Reception**.
- Click on **Policy** to open the office Policy Manual.
- Type "**22**" into the search box to navigate to page 22.
- Read the section of the Policy Manual on the disposal of medications.

1. While checking supplies, Cathy noticed that some of the nonscheduled medications are out of date. These medications are oral tablets and capsules. What means of disposal is correct for these medications?

2. If part of a schedule II medication ampule has to be disposed of, how many clinical medical assistants need to witness the disposal?

 • Click on the exit arrow.
   • Click **Return to Map** and select **Yes** at the pop-up menu to return to the office map or click **Exit the Program**.

Exercise 3

 Writing Activity—Maintaining Administrative Equipment

🕐 10 minutes

1. When filling the copier with paper, Cathy notices that it is time for regular maintenance of the machine and the representative has not been to the office. What should be Cathy's next step?

2. The toner cartridges are low, and Cathy sees a need for replenishing these. What should she do?

Exercise 4

Writing Activity—Suggestions for Equipment and Supplies

10 minutes

1. Ameeta has observed that not all patients with diabetes are using the same glucose meters at home. The physicians are asking that quality control be checked with patients more often. However, if the office does not have the same glucometers and supplies that some of the patients use at home, it is difficult to provide accurate patient teaching. What steps should Ameeta take to ensure that patient teaching is accurate and helpful to each patient?

2. Leah, as an administrative assistant, has found that the phone line for the fax machine is often busy when a fax needs to be received. Often the person attempting to send the fax has called to complain of the difficulty of getting important information to the physicians. What steps should Leah take to show the need for another fax line for the hospital? *Use your critical thinking skills while answering this question.*

Written Communications

📖 **Reading Assignment:** Chapter 13—Written Communication and Document Processing
Chapter 25—Medical Practice Management and Human Resources
- Problem Patients

Patient: Wilson Metcalf

Note: The exercises in this lesson do not specifically involve Wilson Metcalf, but a patient must be selected in order to access the required records.

Learning Objectives:

- Prepare letters in response to the mail received.
- Use correct grammar, spelling, and formatting techniques in letter writing.
- Read mail correspondence correctly.

Overview:

In this lesson you will be asked to respond to incoming mail that includes an NSF check and a letter from a collection agency.

Exercise 1

Online Activity—Composing a Letter for an NSF Check

 40 minutes

- Sign in to Mountain View Clinic.
- Select **Wilson Metcalf** from the patient list.
- Click on **Reception**.
- Click on the **Stackable Trays**.
- Click the numbers or arrows at the top of the page to examine and read each piece of mail.

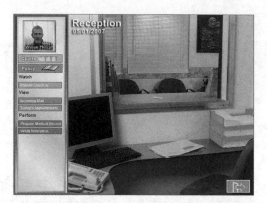

1. Were any payments received in the mail today?

2. List the people from whom payments were received.

3. What is the name of the physician who sent a consultation letter to Dr. Meyer?

4. Who was the letter in reference to?

 • Click the number **7** and read that piece of mail.

5. On the next page, write your letter to the patient about the NSF check, using an acceptable format. Be sure your message conveys the need to handle this matter within a certain number of days and include the charges from the bank in addition to the amount owed the office. Also, include that no further checks will be accepted for this patient's medical care at Mountain View Clinic. This should be prepared for a signature by the office manager.

Mountain View Clinic

4412 Broadway / London, XY 55555 / Phone: (555) 555-1234 / Fax: (555) 555-1239

Nathan Hayler, MD - Family Practice / Katarina Meyer, MD - Internal Medicine

Exercise 2

Online Activity—Composing a Letter in Response to an Inaccurate Accounts Payable

 30 minutes

- Click the number **10** and read that piece of mail.
- From the list of mail at the top of the screen, click on **10** to read the letter from Summer Oxygen Company.
- Click **Finish** to return to the Reception area.
- Click the exit arrow.
- Click **Return to Map** and select **Yes** at the pop-up menu to return to the office map.
- Click on **Office Manager**.
- Click on **Bank Statement** file folder.
- Click on the **Check Ledger** tab.

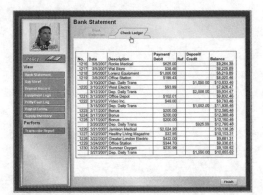

1. There was a payment made to Summer Oxygen Company for $230.99.

    a. According to the check ledger, what was the date the payment was made?

    b. What was the check number?

 • Click on the **Bank Statement** tab to review the account activity for April 2007.

2. Did check #1230 for $230.99 clear the account, according to the bank statement?

3. Below, compose a rough draft for a letter to the Oxygen Supply Company in response to the claim that the invoice has not been paid. Write your letter to the oxygen company using an acceptable format. Be sure your message includes all information needed to clear the accounts payable, and that a copy of the canceled check is enclosed with the letter. This should be prepared for signature by the office manager.

Mountain View Clinic

4412 Broadway / London, XY 55555 / Phone: (555) 555-1234 / Fax (555) 555-1239

Nathan Hayler, MD - Family Practice / Katarina Meyer, MD - Internal Medicine

• Click **Finish** to return to the manager's office.
  • Click the exit arrow.
  • Click **Return to Map** and select **Yes** at the pop-up menu to return to the office map.

Exercise 3

Online Activity—Writing a Termination Letter

 15 minutes

  • Select **Wilson Metcalf** from the patient list.
  • Click on **Reception**.
  • Click on the **Computer**.
  • Scroll down the appointment book to see both the morning and afternoon schedules.

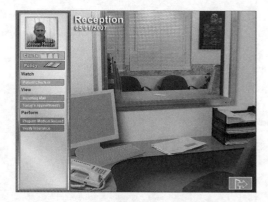

1. What is the name of the patient who has canceled the appointment, and what is the chief complaint?

  • Click **Finish** to return to the Reception area.
  • Click on **Policy** to open the office Policy Manual.
  • Type "cancel" in the search bar and click on the magnifying glass.
  • Read the section of the Policy Manual on canceled appointments.

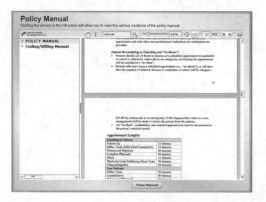

2. Below, compose a letter to the patient you identified in question 1. In the letter, describe the reason for possible termination and the necessary steps needed to remain a patient of Dr. Meyer. The letter should include all of the reasons for possible termination and the need for the patient to keep appointments as made. The letter can also state that Dr. Meyer is concerned about continuity of care and the need for patient safety through this continuity of care.

Mountain View Clinic

4412 Broadway / London, XY 55555 / Phone: (555) 555-1234 / Fax (555) 555-1239

Nathan Hayler, MD - Family Practice / Katarina Meyer, MD - Internal Medicine

3. Why does the letter need to be sent by certified mail?

 4. If a decision is made to terminate a patient, how much time must be allowed between notification and the termination? (*Hint:* Refer to the Problem Patients section in Chapter 25 to answer this question.)

 • Click **Close Manual** to return to the Reception area.
• Click the exit arrow.
• Click **Return to Map**, then click **Yes** at the pop-up menu to return to the office map or click **Exit the Program**.

Organizing a Patient's Medical Record

Reading Assignment: Chapter 11—Patient Reception and Processing
- Registration Procedures

Chapter 14—The Paper Medical Record
- Creating an Efficient Medical Records Management System
- Organization of the Medical Record
- Contents of the Complete Case History
- Making Additions to the Patient Record
- Keeping Records Current
- Filing Procedures (Conditioning)

Chapter 15—The Electronic Medical Record
- Executive Order to Promote Interoperability of EMR Systems
- Technological Terms in Health Information
- American Recovery and Reinvestment Act (ARRA)
- HITECH ACT and Meaningful Use

Patients: Renee Anderson, Tristan Tsosie

Learning Objectives:

- Discuss why proper organization of the medical record is essential.
- Identify and describe the forms found in a medical record.
- Apply principles of medical record organization to choose forms that would be needed when preparing a new patient's medical record.
- Determine whether forms need to be added to the medical record for an established patient.
- Describe the appropriate care of a damaged medical record.
- Determine the appropriate division of medical records when a new record must be established.
- Understand the difference between the terms electronic health record (EHR), electronic medical record (EMR), and personal health record (PHR).
- Identify the goal of EMR interoperability.

Overview:

In this lesson we will explore the importance of preparing a patient's medical record correctly. Because the medical record is a legal document that shows the chronological care of the patient, this document must be correctly organized to ensure that information can be located as needed. Incorrectly organized charts not only cause frustration, but also decrease the efficiency of the medical practice. In this lesson you will organize a medical record for a new patient. For an established patient, you will ensure that information received from other sources has been properly organized and that the information is readily available when the patient arrives for an appointment. You will also be asked to distinguish between the terms *electronic medical record* and *electronic health record*.

Exercise 1

Online Activity—Organizing a Medical Record for a New Patient

 30 minutes

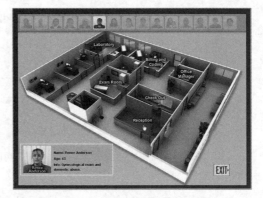

- Sign in to Mountain View Clinic.
- Select **Renee Anderson** from the patient list.
- Click on **Reception**.
- Click on **Policy** to open the Policy Manual.
- Type "medical record" in the search bar and click on the magnifying glass.
- Read the section of the Policy Manual on the duties assigned to the various types of medical assistants in the office.

1. At Mountain View Clinic, the Policy Manual states that the _____ medical assistant is responsible for preparing and organizing the medical record.

Critical Thinking Question

2. Why do you think it is important for the administrative medical assistant to provide the necessary forms in a medical record for a new patient after the patient is "checked" in at the registration desk?

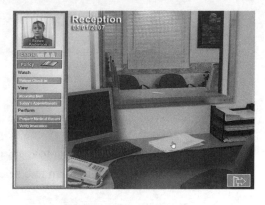

- Click on **Close Manual** to return to the Reception area.
- Click on the **Medical Record**.
- Click on the **Perform** button next to Assemble Medical Record.
- Add forms needed in the Patient Information tab by clicking on the forms from the Forms Available list and clicking **Add** to confirm your choice.
- Make note of all the forms you add into the table below.
- Continue adding forms to the appropriate tabs in the patient's medical record. To select a new tab, either click on the tab on the medical record or use the drop-down menu on the right.
- If you wish to remove a chosen form, highlight the form and click **Remove** at the bottom of the screen.

3. Below, list the forms you added to Renee Anderson's medical record.

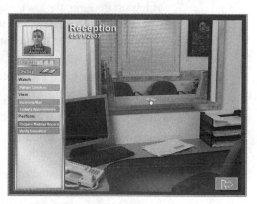

- Click **Finish** to close the chart and return to the Reception area.
- Click on the **Insurance Card**.
- Identify the appropriate question to ask the patient regarding her insurance and click on **Ask**.
- Use the checkboxes to select which procedures are needed to verify the patient's insurance.
- Click **Finish** to return to the Reception area.

4. The form that contains the patient's demographic information is the

   _____.

5. The form in the medical record that contains subjective information about the patient's

   illnesses in the past is the _____.

6. The legal document that must be signed to allow information to be used to file insurance is

   the _____.

7. The form that allows the physician to record findings in the medical record is the

_____.

- Click the exit arrow.
- On the Summary Menu, click on **Look at Your Performance Summary**.
- Scroll down the Performance Summary and compare your answers with those chosen by the experts. The summary can be printed or saved for your instructor.
- Click **Close** to return to the Summary Menu.
- Click **Return to Map** and select **Yes** at the pop-up menu to return to the Office Map.

Exercise 2

Online Activity—Determining Whether to Add Forms to the Medical Record of an Established Patient

 30 minutes

- Select **Tristan Tsosie** from the patient list.
- Click on **Reception**.
- Click on **Charts**.
- Click on the **Hospitalization** tab and select **1-ED Record**.
- Read the ED Record to decide what other forms should be available for the physician for this office visit and to determine whether Tristan is following the orders of the physician who saw him in the Emergency Department. Think about which procedures the patient had while at the Emergency Department and which procedure should have a report to be filed in his chart. Then look under the tabs to see whether you can find the report that you would also need to have available for the physician.

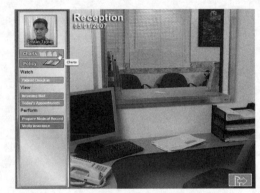

- Click on **Close Chart** to return to the Reception area.

- Click on the **Medical Record**.
- Click on the **Perform** button next to Review and Update Medical Records.
- Review the forms listed under the Patient Information tab. Add any forms that are missing from the Patient Information tab by clicking on the forms from the Forms Available list and clicking **Add** to confirm your choice. The forms you select will appear under the tabs at the bottom of the screen.

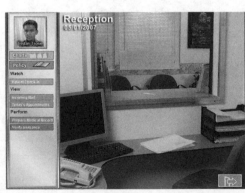

- When you have completed the Patient Information section, continue reviewing and adding forms to the appropriate tabs in Tristan Tsosie's medical record. To select a new tab, either click on the tab on the medical record itself or use the drop-down menu on the right.
- If you wish to remove a chosen form, highlight the form in the tab and click **Remove** at the bottom of the screen.

1. According to the ED Record, with what department was Tristan supposed to follow-up?

2. According to the Consultation Notes, when was Tristan supposed to follow up with the physician? (*Note:* Specify in number of days.)

3. Explain the difference between the terms electronic medical record (EMR) and electronic health records (EHR).

4. If the medical office were sharing information with the hospital, would the record be called EMR or EHR?

5. Did the Emergency Department report advise the patient of when (number of days) to follow up with the doctor? Could this omission of information lead to problems with the patients follow-up care?

6. Other than the ED Record, do any reports related to the ED visit appear in the record? If so, identify the report(s).

7. When adding an abnormal report to the paper medical record, the medical assistant should:
   a. be sure the physician has seen the report before filing it.
   b. place the forms in the medical record in chronological order, with the earliest record on top.
   c. always be sure the date of arrival has been stamped on the report.
   d. wait to file the form just before the patient's arrival for an appointment.
   e. do both a and d.

8. When the medical assistant files materials in the medical record of an established patient, the materials should be filed in what order?

9. When accessing Tristan's medical record on arrival, you notice that the forms from the hospital have been torn during transmittal. What steps do you need to take to maintain the record from further damage?

10. If a patient folder is old, torn, or simply worn, what should the medical assistant do?

11. If a chart is overcrowded and a second chart needs to be established, how far back should the records go that are moved to the new chart? How should the record be marked to show that more than one medical record is available?

12. If the medical office is using an EMR that is interoperable with the hospitals EMR, would the physician have been able to access Tristan's records without having a paper copy in the medical record?

13. What is the goal of EMR interoperability?

14. Who manages, shares, and controls the information in the Personal Health Record (PHR)?

15. What component of the American Recovery and Reimbursement Act (ARRA) awards financial incentives for physicians for using electronic health records.

- Click **Finish** to close the chart and return to the Reception area.
- Click the exit arrow.
- On the Summary Menu, click **Look at Your Performance Summary**.
- Scroll down the Performance Summary to the Patient Records section and compare your answers with those chosen by the experts. The summary can be saved or printed for your instructor.
- Click **Close** to return to the Summary Menu.
- On the Summary Menu, click **Return to Map** and select **Yes** at the pop-up menu to return to the Office Map or click **Exit the Program**.

Exercise 3

Writing Activity—Medical Record Matching Exercise

20 minutes

1. Read the following records and then identify which of the following sections of the medical record each item would be filed in. Write your answer in the lettered blank above each item.

Consent documents
Diagnostic procedure documents
Hospital documents
Medical office administrative documents
Medical office clinical documents
Problem-oriented record
Therapeutic service documents

a. _____

HISTORY AND PHYSICAL
ST. MERCY HOSPITAL

Patient Name: _Carol Jacobs_   Room #: _215_

Physician: _Charles Thomas, MD_   Hospital #: _5422_

Admission Date: _12/14/12_

CHIEF COMPLAINT: Chest pain

HISTORY OF PRESENT ILLNESS: Patient is an 85-year-old female complaining of chest pain. Patient was found to have abnormal cardiac enzymes in the Emergency Room consistent with acute myocardial infarction. Patient denied any pain radiating; however, she did complain of left-sided chest pain and lower back pain. Patient did not admit to any shortness of breath, nausea, or diaphoresis.

MEDICATIONS: Lasix, Darvocet-N 100, Lisinopril, Lopressor, Glynase, Relafen, Cytotec, and Micro K.

ALLERGIES: No drug allergies known.

PAST MEDICAL HISTORY: Significant for congestive heart failure, chronic obstructive pulmonary disease, diabetes mellitus type 2, coronary atherosclerosis, hypertension, and osteoporosis.

SOCIAL HISTORY: Not a drinker and not a smoker. Patient resides in a nursing home.

PHYSICAL EXAMINATION:

General: Patient is in acute distress. She is obese.

HEENT: She has 2 centimeters jugular venous distention. Pupils are equal and reactive to light and accommodation. No evidence of scleral or conjunctival icterus.

Chest: +2 bibasilar rales.

Heart: Regular rate and rhythm. +2/6 systolic ejection murmur in the left sternal border.

Abdomen: Soft, nontender, no splenomegaly and no hepatomegaly and positive bowel sounds.

Extremities: No evidence of edema or deep venous thrombosis.

Neurological: Cranial nerves II through XII grossly intact.

IMPRESSIONS: Congestive heart failure
                          Rule out myocardial infarction

Charles Thomas, MD

Charles Thomas, MD

b. _____

COLLEGE HOSPITAL
4567 BROAD AVENUE
WOODLAND HILLS, MD 21532

RADIOLOGY REPORT

Examination Date:	June 14, 2012	Patient:	Rose Baker
Date Reported:	June 14, 2012	X-ray No.:	43200
Physician:	Harold B. Cooper, M.D.	Age:	19
Examination:	PA Chest, Abdomen	Hospital No.:	80-32-11

FINDINGS

PA CHEST: Upright PA view of chest shows the lung fields are clear, without evidence of an active process. Heart size is normal. There is no evidence of pneumoperitoneum.

IMPRESSION: NEGATIVE CHEST

ABDOMEN: Flat and upright views of the abdomen show a normal gas pattern without evidence of obstruction or ileus. There are no calcifications or abnormal masses noted.

IMPRESSION: NEGATIVE STUDY

RADIOLOGIST: _Marian B. Skinner_

Marian B. Skinner, MD

c. _____

DISCHARGE SUMMARY

Brennan, Susan
97-32-11
June 18, 2012

ADMISSION DATE: June 14, 2012   **DISCHARGE DATE:**   June 16, 2012

HISTORY OF PRESENT ILLNESS:
This 19-year-old female, nulligravida, was admitted to the hospital on June 14, 2012, with fever of 102°, left lower quadrant pain, vaginal discharge, constipation, and a tender left adnexal mass. Her past history and family history were unremarkable. Present pain had started two to three weeks prior to admission. Her periods were irregular, with latest period starting on May 30, 2012, and lasting for six days. She had taken contraceptive pills in the past but had stopped because she was not sexually active.

PHYSICAL EXAMINATION:
She appeared well developed and well nourished, and in mild distress. The only positive physical findings were limited to the abdomen and pelvis. Her abdomen was mildly distended, and it was tender, especially in the left lower quadrant. At pelvic examination, her cervix was tender on motion, and the uterus was of normal size, retroverted, and somewhat fixed. There was a tender cystic mass about 4-5 cm in the left adnexa. Rectal examination was negative.

PROVISIONAL DIAGNOSIS:
1. Probable pelvic inflammatory disease (PID).
2. Rule out ectopic pregnancy.

LABORATORY DATA ON ADMISSION:
Hgb 10.8, Hct 36.5, WBC 8,100 with 80 segs and 18 lymphs. Sedimentation rate 100 mm in one hour. Sickle cell prep+ (turned out to be a trait). Urinalysis normal. Electrolytes normal. SMA-12 normal. Chest x-ray negative, 2-hour UCG negative.

HOSPITAL COURSE AND TREATMENT:
Initially, she was given cephalothin 2 gm IV q6h, and kanamycin 0.5 gm IM bid. Over the next two days the patient's condition improved. Her pain decreased and her temperature came down to normal in the morning and spiked to 101° in the evening. Repeat CBC showed Hgb 9.8, Hct 33.5. The pregnancy test was negative. She was discharged on June 16, 2012 in good condition. She will be seen in the office in one week.

DISCHARGE DIAGNOSIS:
Pelvic inflammatory disease.

Harold B. Cooper, MD
Harold B. Cooper, MD

d. _____

EMERGENCY DEPARTMENT REPORT
CAMDEN CLARK HOSPITAL

Name: John Larimer   DOB: 2/2/72

ER Physician: John Parsons, MD   Date: 7/7/12

ER Number: 07398

Physician: James Woods, MD

NATURE OF ILLNESS/INJURY: This 40-year-old male presents to the Emergency Department complaining of a laceration of the sole of his right foot. Patient cut his foot on a rock 2 days ago and thinks he might have an infection now. Patient also complains of coughing over the past several days.

PHYSICAL EXAMINATION: Temperature 97.4, Pulse 76, Respirations 20, Blood Pressure 120/70. Patient is alert and oriented and is in no acute distress. ENT is normal. Lungs show diffuse rhonchi without crackles or wheezing. Heart has a regular rate and rhythm. Right great toe with marked tenderness with edema and erythema and heat.

DIAGNOSIS: Asthmatic Bronchitis
        Cellulitis, right foot first MTP

TREATMENT: PCMX scrub to right foot. Bacitracin dressing. Tetanus Diphtheria 0.5 cc IM. Biaxin 500 mg bid x 10 days. Guaifenesin with codeine 2 tsp q4h prn. Entex LA,1 bid prn. Debridement of skin flap.

PATIENT INSTRUCTIONS: Patient to follow up with family doctor in 7 days. Discussed bronchospasms with the patient.

James Woods, MD

James Woods, MD

e. _____

(Attach label or complete blanks.)

First name: _____   Last name: _____

Date of Birth: _____ Month _____ Day _____ Year

Account Number: _____

Procedure Consent Form

I, _____ , hereby consent to have

Dr. _____   perform _____ .

I have been fully informed of the following by my physician:

1. The nature of my condition
2. The nature and purpose of the procedure
3. An explanation of risks involved with the procedure
4. Alternative treatments or procedures available
5. The likely results of the procedure
6. The risks involved with declining or delaying the procedure

My physician has offered to answer all questions concerning the proposed procedure.

I am aware that the practice of medicine and surgery is not an exact science, and I acknowledge that no guarantees have been made to me about the results of the procedure.

Patient _____   Date _____
          (or guardian and relationship)

Witnessed _____   Date _____

f. _____

PROBLEM ORIENTED - PROGRESS NOTES

Date	Time	Problem Number	FORMAT:	Problem Number and TITLE: S = Subjective	O = Objective	A = Assessment	P = Plan
11/15/12	9:30 AM	1	S:	Mother states that her child has had a runny nose and her throat has been			
				sore for 2 days.			
			O:	Vital signs: T 98.8 P 96 R 24			
				Weight: 42 lb.			
				General: alert and active. HEENT: sclera clear. TMs negative. Positive clear			
				rhinorrhea. Pharynx benign. Heart: regular without murmur.			
				Lungs: clear to auscultation and percussion. Abdomen: negative tenderness.			
				Positive bowel x 4. GU: negative. Neuro: good tone.			
			A:	Upper respiratory tract infection.			
			P:	1. A prescription for Rondec DM, 1/2 tsp q6h prn cough and congestion.			
				2. Instructed mother to contact office if child does not improve.			

NAME-Last	First	Middle	Attending Physician	Record No.	Room/Bed
Michaels	Jessica	L	Frank Edwards, MD	1	24

Form 689/35 ©BRIGGS, Des Moines, IA 50306 (800) 247-2343 www.BriggsCorp.com
PRINTED IN U.S.A.

PROBLEM ORIENTED - PROGRESS NOTES

g. _____

OPERATIVE REPORT
ST. MARY'S HOSPITAL

Name: Natalie Boyer

Hospital #: 291734   Room #: OP

Surgeon: Paul Cain, M.D.   Date of Surgery: 1/6/12

Assistants: N/A   Anesthesia: General

Anesthesiologist: John Adams, M.D.

PRE-OP DIAGNOSIS: Abnormal Pap test with history of cervical carcinoma.

POST-OP DIAGNOSIS: Same and awaiting path report.

PROCEDURE: D&C, laser cone of the cervix.

The patient to the operating room, lithotomy position, perineum and vagina were prepped, and moist sterile drape was used. Laser precautions all in place. Bimanual examination revealed a uterus enlarged with a second-degree uterine prolapse. The cervix was dilated. Uterus sounded to around 9 cm. The endocervical canal was dilated and D&C was performed with tissue recovered and submitted to Pathology. The cervix was stained with iodine, and the nonstaining area was identified. The laser was brought in, 50 watts of current were used to remove laser cone, and we submitted that to Pathology. We then vaporized beyond the margins of the cone, 3-4 mm to a depth of 4-5 mm. Hemostasis was adequate. We placed 0 Vicryl figure-of-eight sutures at the 3 and the 9 o'clock positions in the cervix, and then we put Monsel solution on the cervix. Hemostasis adequate. Sponge and needle counts correct times two. The patient tolerated the procedure well, and she returned to the recovery room in stable condition. She will be discharged home when awake and stable on Cipro 250 mg twice a day for a week, Darvocet-N 100, #20 as needed for pain. If she continues to have abnormal Pap tests, we will probably want to do a vaginal hysterectomy.

SURGEON: _Paul Cain, MD_
          Paul Cain, MD

h. _____

HAROLD B. COOPER, M.D.
6000 MAIN STREET
VENTURA, CA 93003

June 15, 2012

John F. Millstone, M.D.
5302 Main Street
Ventura, CA 93003

Dear Dr. Millstone:

RE: Elaine J. Silverman

This 69-year-old woman was seen at your request. The patient was admitted to the hospital yesterday because of chills, fever, and abdominal and back pain.

REVIEW OF HEALTH HISTORY: The history has been reviewed. A prominent feature of the history is the presence of intermittent, severe, shaking chills for four days with associated left lower back pain, left lower quadrant abdominal pain, and fever to as high as 103 or 104 degrees. The patient has had hypertension for a number of years and has been managed quite well with Aldomet 250 mg twice a day.

PHYSICAL EXAMINATION: On examination her temperature at this time is 100.6 degrees. The pulse is 110 and regular. Blood pressure is 190/100. The patient has partial bilateral iridectomies, the result of previous cataract surgery. Otherwise, the head and neck are not remarkable. Lung fields are clear throughout. The heart reveals a regular tachycardia, and heart sounds are of good quality. No murmurs are heard, and there is no gallop rhythm present. The abdomen is soft. There is no spasm or guarding. A well-healed surgical scar is present in the right flank area. There is considerable tenderness in the left lower quadrant of the left mid abdomen, but as noted, there is no spasm or guarding present. Bowel sounds are present. Peristaltic rushes are noted, and the bowel sounds are slightly high pitched. The extremities are unremarkable.

IMPRESSIONS: I believe the patient has acute diverticulitis. She may have some irritation of the left ureter in view of the findings on the urinalysis. She appears to be responding to therapy at this time in that her temperature is coming down and there has been a slight reduction in the leukocytosis from yesterday.

RECOMMENDATIONS: I agree with the present program of therapy, and the only suggestion would be to possibly increase the dose of gentamicin to 60 mg q8h, rather than the 40 mg q8h that she is now receiving.

Thank you for asking me to see this patient in consultation.

Sincerely,

Harold B. Cooper

Harold B. Cooper, M.D.

mtf

---

i. _____

PHYSICAL THERAPY EVALUATION

OBJECTIVE DATA TESTS AND SCALES PRINTED ON REVERSE.

DATE OF SERVICE 9 / 23 / 12

HOMEBOUND REASON: ☐ Needs assistance for all activities ☐ Residual weakness
☐ Requires assistance to ambulate ☐ Confusion, unable to go out of home alone
☐ Unable to safely leave home unassisted ☐ Severe SOB, SOB upon exertion
☐ Dependent upon adaptive device(s) ☐ Medical restrictions
☐ Other (specify)_____

SOC DATE 9 / 23 / 12
[If Initial Evaluation, complete Physical Therapy Care Plan]

PERTINENT BACKGROUND INFORMATION

OTHER DISCIPLINES PROVIDING CARE: ☐ SN ☐ OT ☐ ST ☐ MSW ☐ Aide

MEDICAL HISTORY
☐ Hypertension ☐ Cancer
☐ Cardiac ☐ Infection
☐ Diabetes ☐ Immunosuppressed
☐ Respiratory ☐ Open wound
☐ Osteoporosis ☐ Falls with injury
☐ Fractures ☐ Falls without injury
☐ Other (specify)_____

REASON FOR EVALUATION (Diagnosis/Problem)
Hx Ⓛ knee pain x 5 yrs, little relief c̄ PT
_____
_____
_____
_____
_____

LIVING SITUATION
☒ Capable ☐ Able ☐ Willing caregiver available
☐ Limited caregiver support (ability/willingness)
☐ No caregiver available
HOME SAFETY BARRIERS:
☐ Clutter ☐ Throw rugs ☐ Bath bench/equipment ☐ Needs grab bar
☐ Needs railings ☐ Steps (number/condition)_____
☐ Other (specify)_____

PRIOR LEVEL OF FUNCTION
ADLs:
☒ Independent ☐ Needed assistance ☐ Unable
Equipment used:_____

IN-HOME MOBILITY (gait or wheelchair/scooter):
☒ Independent ☐ Needed assistance ☐ Unable
Equipment used:_____

COMMUNITY MOBILITY (gait or wheelchair/scooter):
☐ Independent ☐ Needed assistance ☐ Unable
Equipment used:_____

BEHAVIOR/MENTAL STATUS
☒ Alert ☐ Oriented ☐ Cooperative ☐ Confused ☐ Memory deficits
☐ Impaired judgement ☐ Other (specify)_____

VITAL SIGNS/CURRENT STATUS
Blood Pressure:_____
Temperature:_____
Pulse:_____
Respirations:_____
O₂ saturation _____ % (when ordered): ☐ at rest ☐ with activity
Skin:_____
Edema:_____
Vision: _glasses_____
Sensation:_____
Communication:_____
Hearing:_____
Posture:_____
Endurance:_____

PAIN
INTENSITY: 0 1 2 3 4 ⑤ 6 7 8 9 10
LOCATION:_____
AGGRAVATING FACTORS:_____
_____
RELIEVING FACTORS:_____
_____
BEST PAIN GETS: _2_   WORST PAIN GETS: _8_
ACCEPTABLE LEVEL OF PAIN:_____
CURRENT LEVEL OF PAIN:_____
IMPACT ON THERAPY POC? ☐ None ☐ (describe)_____
_____
_____

PATIENT NAME = Last, First, Middle Initial
Johnson, Thomas, J.

ID#

Form 3841P © Briggs, Des Moines, IA 50306 (800) 247-2343 www.BriggsCorp.com

PHYSICAL THERAPY EVALUATION
☐ Continued on Reverse

j. _____

RELEASE OF MEDICAL INFORMATION

All information contained in the medical record is confidential, and the release of information is closely controlled. A properly completed and signed authorization form is required for the release of the following information.

PATIENT INFORMATION

Patient Name _____

Address _____ Social Security # _____

City _____ State _____ ZIP _____ Birth date ____/____/____

Phone (Home) _____ Work _____

RELEASE FROM:

Name _____

Address _____

City _____ State _____ ZIP _____

RELEASE TO:

Name _____

Address _____

City _____ State _____ ZIP _____

INFORMATION TO BE RELEASED:

1. GENERAL RELEASE:

____ Entire Medical Record (excluding protected information)

____ Hospital Records only (specify) _____

____ Lab Results only (specify) _____

____ X-ray Reports only (specify) _____

____ Other Records (specify) _____

2. INFORMATION PROTECTED BY STATE/FEDERAL LAW:
If indicated below, I hereby authorize the disclosure and release of information regarding:

____ Drug Abuse Diagnosis/Treatment

____ Alcoholism Diagnosis/Treatment

____ Mental Health Diagnosis/Treatment

____ Sexually Transmitted Disease

PURPOSE/NEED FOR INFORMATION:

____ Taking records to another doctor

____ Moving

____ Legal purposes

____ Insurance purposes

____ Worker's Compensation

____ Other/Explain: _____

METHOD OF RELEASE:

____ US Mail

____ Fax

____ Telephone

____ To Patient

PATIENT AUTHORIZATION TO RELEASE INFORMATION:

Authorization is valid for 60 days only from the date of my signature. I reserve the right to revoke this authorization at any time prior to 60 days (except for action that has already been taken) by notifying the medical office in writing.

I understand that my records are protected under HIPAA (Health Insurance Portability and Accountability Act) Standards for Privacy of Individually Identifiable Information (45 CFR Parts 160 and 164) unless otherwise permitted by federal law. Any information released or received shall not be further relayed to any other facility or person without my written authorization. I also understand that such information will not be given, sold, transferred, or in any way relayed to any other person or party not specified above without my further written authorization.

I hereby grant authorization to release the information listed above. I certify that this request has been made voluntarily and that the information given above is accurate to the best of my knowledge.

_____ _____

Signature of Patient/Legally Responsible Party   Date

_____ _____

Witness Signature   Date

OFFICE USE ONLY

Information indicated above released on _____
                                              Date

Explanation of information released: _____

_____

Signature and credentials of individual releasing information: _____

k. _____

PATIENT INFORMATION	CONFIDENTIAL		File no. 10140

(PLEASE PRINT)

Date 11-21-12

Name Carol H Jones   Birth date 1-20-68   Home phone 740-555-1248
First Middle Last

Address 743 Evergreen Terrace   City Springfield   State OH   ZIP 12345

Check appropriate box: ☐ Minor ☐ Single ☒ Married ☐ Divorced ☐ Widowed ☐ Separated   Gender: ☐ Male ☒ Female

Employer Rockford, Inc.   Work phone 740-555-1234

Business address 1 Rockford Place   City Shelbyville   State OH   ZIP 21346

Spouse or parent's name John Jones   Employer Self-emp.   Work phone 740-555-8654

If patient is a student, name of school/college N/A   City _____ State _____

Whom may we thank for referring you? Henry Peterson, MD

Person to contact in case of emergency John Jones   Phone 740-555-1248

RESPONSIBLE PARTY

Name of person responsible for this account Carol Jones   Relationship to patient Self

Address 743 Evergreen Terrace   City Springfield   State OH   ZIP 12345   Home phone 740-555-1248

Employer Rockford, Inc.   Work phone 740-555-1234

Is this person currently a patient in our office?   ☒ Yes   ☐ No

INSURANCE INFORMATION

Name of insured Carol Jones   Relationship to patient Self

Birth date 1-20-68   Social Security number 123-45-6789   Date employed 5-1-93

Name of employer Rockford, Inc.   Work phone 740-555-1234

Address of employer 1 Rockford Place   City Shelbyville   State OH   ZIP 21346

Insurance company Anthem BC/BS   Group number 51045

Insurance company address 521 Anthem Drive   City New Haberville   State OH   ZIP 21436

DO YOU HAVE ANY ADDITIONAL INSURANCE?   ☐ YES   ☒ NO   IF YES, COMPLETE THE FOLLOWING:

Name of insured _____   Relationship to patient _____

Birth date _____   Social Security number _____   Date employed _____

Name of employer _____   Work phone _____

Address of employer _____   City _____   State _____ ZIP _____

Insurance company _____   Group number _____

Insurance company address _____   City _____   State _____ ZIP _____

X *Carol Jones*
SIGNATURE OF PATIENT OR PARENT IF MINOR

1. _____

DIAGNOSTIC IMAGING REPORT			
Mt. Carmel Hospital, Columbus, OH 43201			
DATE REQUESTED 6/6/2012	DATE TO BE DONE 6/10/2012	TODAY'S DATE 6/10/2012	DATE OF BIRTH 8/19/1949
☐ WHEELCHAIR	☐ PORTABLE	☒ AMBULATORY	☐ CART

PATIENT: Vera Ruth **INSURANCE:** Industrial

SEX F	ROOM NO. OP	RESPONSIBLE PERSON OR EMPLOYER J.B. Warren, Inc.	RADIOLOGIST Richard W. Adams, MD

CLINICAL INFORMATION AND PROVISIONAL DIAGNOSIS

Back injury

ATTENDING PHYSICIAN Christopher Robb, MD

NURSE

EXAMINATION REQUESTED (PINPOINT AREA OF CONCERN IF POSSIBLE)

CT LUMBAR SPINE

TECHNIQUE:

CT of the lumbar spine without contrast was performed from L-3 through S-1.

FINDINGS:

The L3-4 level appears satisfactory without evidence of osseous proliferation or disc protrusion.

At the L4-5 level there is some increased density at the disc level, which may be more prominent on the left. This is partially obscured due to facet artifact crossing obliquely.

There does appear to be some retention of epidural fat plane. This, however, may represent left-sided disc bulge or protrusion with the appropriate corresponding clinical appearance. Osseous variation at this level is not identified.

At the L5-S1 level, significant variation is not apparent.

IMPRESSION:

Variation at the L4-5 level on the left, which may represent annular disc bulge or perhaps protrusion on the left. However, confirmation with myelography and/or Ampaque enhanced computed tomography of the lumbar spine should be suggested prior to any surgical intervention.

Richard W. Adams, MD

Richard W. Adams, MD

m. _____

COLLEGE HOSPITAL
4567 BROAD AVENUE
WOODLAND HILLS, MD 21532

PATHOLOGY REPORT

Date:	June 20, 2012	Pathology No.:	430211
Patient:	Molly Ramsdale	Room No.:	1308
Physician:	Harold B. Cooper, M.D.		
Specimen Submitted:	Tumor, right axilla		

FINDINGS

GROSS DESCRIPTION: Specimen A consists of an oval mass of yellow fibroadipose tissue measuring 4 x 3 x 2 cm. On cut section, there are some small, soft, pliable areas of gray apparent lymph node alternating with adipose tissue. A frozen section consultation at time of surgery was delivered as NO EVIDENCE OF MALIGNANCY on frozen section, to await permanent section for final diagnosis. Majority of the specimen will be submitted for microscopic examination.

Specimen B consists of an oval mass of yellow soft tissue measuring 2.5 x 2.5 x 1.5 cm. On cut section, there is a thin rim of pink to tan-brown lymphatic tissue and the mid portion appears to be adipose tissue. A pathological consultation at time of surgery was delivered as no suspicious areas noted and to await permanent sections for final diagnosis. The entire specimen will be submitted for microscopic examination.

MICROSCOPIC DESCRIPTION: Specimen A sections show fibroadipose tissue and nine fragments of lymph nodes. The lymph nodes show areas with prominent germinal centers and moderate sinus histiocytosis. There appears to be some increased vascularity and reactive endothelial cells seen. There is no evidence of malignancy.

Specimen B sections show adipose tissue and 5 lymph node fragments. These 5 portions of lymph nodes show reactive changes including sinus histiocytosis. There is no evidence of malignancy.

DIAGNOSIS: A & B: TUMOR, RIGHT AXILLA: SHOWING 14 LYMPH NODE FRAGMENTS WITH REACTIVE CHANGES AND NO EVIDENCE OF MALIGNANCY.

Stanley T. Nason, MD

Stanley T. Nason, MD

n. _____

PATIENT RECORD

Name	Morani, Betty				ALLERGIES/SENSITIVITY				
Number		Blood Type: A+			Codeine, Sulfa				

Prob. No.	Date	PROBLEM DESCRIPTION	Date Resolved	Index	Prob. No.	Date	PROBLEM DESCRIPTION	Date Resolved	Index
1	10/05	Hypertension - essential		✓					
2	10/05	Diabetes mellitus (mild)		✓					
3	1/08	L. Retinopathy _ _ _ _ _	see below						
4	4/2012	Atherosclerosis with cerebral vascular insuffic.							
5	4/2012	Hearing loss							
6	1/2012	HBP Non-compliance	2/12						
3	1/2012	Bilat. Grade II Retinopathy							

Prob. No.	CONTINUING MEDICATIONS	Start	Stop	Prob. No.	CONTINUING MEDICATIONS	Start	Stop
1	Sinoserp 1 mg. b.i.d.	10/05	10/09				
2	Orinase 0.5 gm. daily	10/05	10/09				
1	Hydrodiuril 50 mg. A.M.	10/05					
2	1500 cal. diet low Na hi K	2/2012					

Periodic Health Examination	Dates	1/04	4/06	2/08	1/10							

o. _____

Form 2014/2 (5 2-part set) or	BRIGGS, Des Moines, IA 50306 (800) 247-2343
Form 2014/3 (5 3-part set)	PRINTED IN U.S.A.

Home Health Agency — Visit Report

Date of Visit	11/21/12	Start: 7	Mileage	Finish: 9

Patient's Name Clarence Casker

Financial:		Med. A:	Med. B:
GH:	VA:	Pvt	Other: Hospice

BP (L): 160/82	(R): 160/82	T: 97.7	Area:	Diagnosis: Lung Cancer

P (A): 78	(R): 76	Wt: 151	R: 18	Procedure:	Age: 74

Pt. Instruction: Continue O₂ as needed

Comments/Observations: (Physical, mental, emotional, activity level, Environ., S/S, Treatments & Effects, Procedures, Med. Effects, Other)

Pt complaining of some difficulty breathing and swelling of his feet. Pt was given Provehtil Atrovent neb tx

and started on oxygen at 2 liters per nasal canula. Tx was discussed with Dr. Shay.

Plan: Monitor vitals every 2 hrs.

Supplies Used: O₂ @ 2 liters

Signature: D. Talley, RN

Next Visit:	11/22/12	RN ✓	PT	HHA	MSW	Other
Freq. of Visits:	Daily	✓				
Travel Time:			Service Time:			

Supervisory Visit:

Form 20P14   © BRIGGS, Des Moines, IA 50306 (800) 247-2343   PRINTED IN U.S.A.

Filing Medical Records

Reading Assignment: Chapter 14—The Paper Medical Record
- Creating an Efficient Medical Records Management System
- Filing Procedures
- Filing Methods
- Organization of Files

Chapter 15—The Electronic Medical Record
- Technological Terms in Health Information
- Capabilities of EMR Systems

Patients: All

Learning Objectives:

- Alphabetize patient names for efficiency in filing medical records.
- List the necessary steps needed to prepare a paper medical record for filing.
- Describe the use of color coding to enhance paper medical record systems.
- Identify the filing systems used most frequently in the medical office for patient records.
- Discuss the differences between alphabetic and numeric filing systems.
- Determine which patients are established patients and which are new patients for preparing charts.
- Discuss the means for finding displaced paper medical records.
- Explain the most important function of primary features that EMR software may offer.

Overview:

Proper filing of medical records is essential in providing continuity of care for patients. You will determine if patients are new or established in preparation for filing and you will then alphabetize patients. You will be asked to differentiate between alphabetic and numeric filing systems and identify methods for locating misplaced medical information. One activity will involve answering questions about the different features with which typical EMR software comes.

Exercise 1

Online Activity—Preparing Patient Medical Records for Filing

 50 minutes

- Sign in to Mountain View Clinic.
- Select **Janet Jones** from the patient list.
- Click on **Reception**.
- Click on the **Computer**.
- Scroll down the appointment book to see both the morning and afternoon schedules.

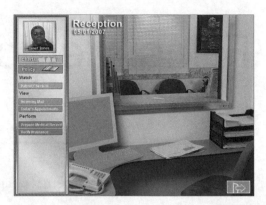

1. Look for each patient's name and note next to his or her name on the table above whether that patient is a new patient (NP) or an established patient (Est. Pt.) (*Note:* You will return to fill in the remaining columns of the table later in this exercise.)

Patient Name	New Patient (NP) or Established Patient (Est. Pt.)	First Date of Service mm/dd/yy	Last Date of Service mm/dd/yy
Janet Jones			
Wilson Metcalf			
Rhea Davison			
Shaunti Begay			
Jean Deere			
Renee Anderson			
Teresa Hernandez			
Louise Parlet			
Tristan Tsosie			
Jose Imero			
Jade Wong			
John R. Simmons			
Hu Huang			
Kevin McKinzie			
Jesus Santo			

2. With the schedule of Today's Appointments still open, make a list below of the patients Dr. Hayler is to see in the morning. Place these patients in the correct order for their appointments and note whether the medical record can be pulled from the files of established patients or whether a new record should be prepared.

3. What medical records will need to be pulled from the files for Dr. Meyer's morning patients? Will any of these patients need to have a new record prepared? List these patients and their record needs below (in the order of their appointment times).

 • Click **Finish** to return to the Reception area.

• Click on **Charts**.

• Click on the **Patient Medical Information** tab and select **1-Progress Notes**.

• Record the patient's first and last dates of service in columns 3 and 4 in the table in question 1. (*Important:* New patients will not have any forms in their chart. Use today's virtual date—5/1/07—as their first date of service; there will be no "last date of service" for new patients.)

• Click **Close Chart** to return to the Reception area.

• Click the exit arrow.

• Click **Return to Map** and select **Yes** at the pop-up menu to return to the office map.

• Repeat these instructions for each patient until you have completed the table in question 1.

4. Using the table in question 1 as a reference, list the patients' names in alphabetic order in the left column below. In the right column indicate whether the medical records for each patient will be available in the file cabinet of established patients or whether the record will have to be organized and placed in the correct position as a new medical record.

Alphabetic List of Patients	New or Established Record?

5. As you pull the medical records for established patients, you will need to change the year on the medical records for these patients (unless the patient has already been seen in the current year). List the established patients below and indicate what year will need to be relabeled on their medical record (if this applies). Remember, today's virtual date is May 1, 2007.

Name of Established Patient	Year That Will Need to Be Relabeled

6. At the end of the morning, the medical records need to be filed correctly to prevent loss and to ensure proper time management. Below, list in alphabetic order the names of patients who had morning appointments today and whose records will need to be refiled.

 • Click the exit arrow.
• Click **Return to Map**, then click **Yes** at the pop-up menu to return to the office map or click Exit the Program.

Exercise 2

 Writing Activity

 25 minutes

Answer the following questions regarding paper medical records and capabilities of EMR systems.

1. Which of the following would *not* be used to help prevent misfiling of medical records?
   a. Colored letter tabs for use with names
   b. Colored tabs for the last year seen in the office
   c. Outguides
   d. Alphabetic tabs in the filing system

2. The two filing systems most often used in a medical office are

   _____ and _____ filing.

3. Describe the differences in alphabetic and numeric filing systems.

4. Explain how color-coding enhances paper medical record systems?

5. List the five steps needed to prepare a paper medical record for filing.

(1)

(2)

(3)

(4)

(5)

6. What steps can be followed for "finding" a misplaced paper medical record?

7. Explain the primary function of the following features of EMR software systems.

   a. Specialty software

   b. Appointment scheduler

   c. Appointment reminder and confirmation

   d. Prescription writer

   e. Medical billing systems

f. Charge capture

g. Eligibility verification

h. Referral management

i. Laboratory order integration

j. Patient portal

Insurance Forms and Verification

Reading Assignment: Chapter 7—Medicine and Law
- OSHA Record Keeping Regulations

Chapter 18—Basics of Diagnostic Coding

Chapter 19—Basics of Procedural Coding

Chapter 20—Basics of Health Insurance

Chapter 21—The Health Insurance Claim Form

Patients: Shaunti Begay, Louise Parlet, John R. Simmons, Janet Jones, Jose Imero

Learning Objectives:

- Apply managed care policies and procedures to office billing and coding.
- Use third party guidelines for preparing insurance claims and collecting copayments.
- Verify insurance information and initiate a referral for a patient.
- Determine which diagnosis should be coded, and which should not, from patient documentation in the chart.
- Proofread an insurance claim form and identify errors that will affect claims processing.

Overview:

In this lesson you will perform the necessary steps for preparing a clean claim for insurance purposes and collecting co-payments that are due to the practice. Completing these steps requires the correct use of managed care policies and procedures and the proper application of the office Policy Manual. A clean claim includes the appropriate diagnostic and procedural codes as well as the proper completion of the insurance claim form. You will proofread an insurance form and compare it with the information in the patient's chart and encounter form. You will indicate which boxes need corrections before the claim can be sent to the insurance company.

Exercise 1

 Online Activity—Verifying Insurance for a New Patient

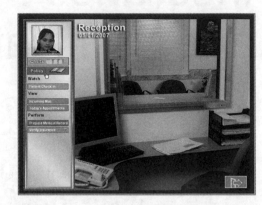

🕐 30 minutes

- Sign in to Mountain View Clinic.
- Select **Shaunti Begay** from the patient list.
- Click on **Reception**.
- Click on **Policy** to open the office Policy Manual.
- Type "payment" in the search bar and click on the magnifying glass.
- Read the section of the Policy Manual on the Telephone Policies, specifically concerning copays.
- Type "patient insurance policies" in the search bar and click on the magnifying glass.
- Read the section of the Policy Manual on the policies that apply when patients have insurance coverage that is not accepted by the medical practice.

1. According to the Policy Manual, what information should be obtained from the patient when the appointment is made?

   All information to complete forms

2. Why is it important for the medical assistant to verify whether the office is a preferred provider with the patient's insurance *at the time the appointment is made*?

   Prevent misunderstandings
   Ensure payment

3. What does the Policy Manual state about collecting payments, copays, and percentages of charges for patient visits?

   Collect at time of service, patient must be told during scheduling

- Click **Close Manual** to return to the Reception desk.
- Under the Watch heading, click on **Patient Check-In** and watch the video.
- Click the **X** on the video screen to close the video.
- Click on the **Insurance Card**.
- Identify the appropriate question to ask the patient regarding her insurance and click on **Ask**.
- Use the checkboxes to select which procedures are needed to verify the patient's insurance.
- Click **Finish** to return to the Reception area.

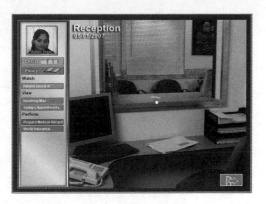

- Click on **Policy** to open the office Policy Manual.
- From the menu on the left side of the screen, click on the arrow next to **Coding/Billing Manual** to expand the menu.
- Click the arrow next to **Financial Policy** and select **Accepted Insurance Carriers** from the list to read that section of the Policy Manual.

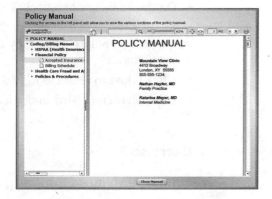

4. Was Kristin correct in stating that Mountain View Clinic was not a participating provider for Shaunti's insurance plan?

Yes

5. What did Shaunti's mother say about the information she gave the receptionist regarding their insurance coverage when she made the appointment?

Didn't know which plan when they made the appointment

6. What steps should the medical assistant have taken to avoid the confusion that occurred when Shaunti checked in?

Ask mother to first find the name of the insurance before scheduling

→ • Click **Close Manual** to return to the Reception area.
   • Click the exit arrow.
   • On the Summary Menu, click on **Look at Your Performance Summary**.
   • Scroll down the Performance Summary to the Verify Insurance section and compare your answers with those chosen by the experts. The summary can be printed or saved for your instructor.
   • Click **Close** to return to the Summary Menu.
   • Click **Return to Map** and select **Yes** at the pop-up menu to return to the office map.

Exercise 2

Online Activity—Obtaining a Referral for an Established Patient

 30 minutes

   • Select **Louise Parlet** from the patient list.
   • Click on **Check Out**.
   • Under the Watch heading, click on **Patient Check-Out** and watch the video.

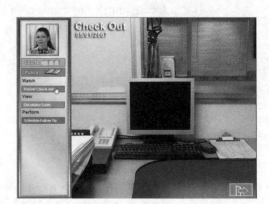

1. Why is it important that the medical assistant assist Ms. Parlet in obtaining approval from her insurance company for the referral to Dr. Lockett?

Need to get ASAP Appointment in 3 days

2. After receiving the precertification verification number, how should the medical assistant handle the verification number?

document and saved to specialist

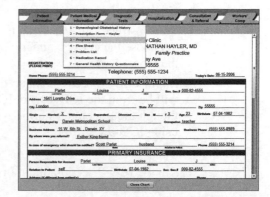

- Click the **X** on the video screen to close the video.
- Click on **Charts**.
- Click on the **Patient Medical Information** tab and select **3-Progress Notes**.
- Read Dr. Hayler's notes regarding the examination.

3. What instructions does Dr. Hayler give about the results of the lab work?

Copy   Sent to OB

Critical Thinking Question

4. Do you think most insurance companies would reimburse a medical provider for a test if the test has already been completed at another facility?

yes/no

- Click **Close Chart** to return to the Check Out desk.
- Click the exit arrow.
- Click **Return to Map** and select **Yes** at the pop-up menu to return to the office map.

Exercise 3

Online Activity—Choosing the Correct Diagnosis to Code for an Office Visit of a New Adult Patient

🕐 30 minutes

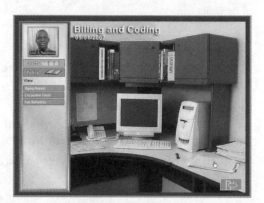

- Select **John R. Simmons** from the patient list.
- Click on **Billing and Coding**.
- Click on the **Encounter Form** clipboard.
- Your instructor may ask you to use the ICD-10 to choose the correct numeric codes for the diagnoses listed.
- *Important:* Please remember that your codes will be from the ICD-10, not ICD-9, even though the Encounter Form says the clinic is using ICD-9.

1. In the ICD-9 section of the Encounter Form, which diagnoses are checked off for Dr. Simmons' visit?

   * headache
   * hematuria
   * hypertension
     ↑ BP

2. Which of these diagnoses should receive an ICD-9 code? If there are any diagnoses that should not be coded, explain why not.

3. When should the fecal occult Hemoccult test that the patient will collect at home be billed? Explain your answer.

   When test cards are returned and developed. Don't bill for tests that aren't completed

- Click **Finish** to return to the Billing and Coding area.
- Click on **Charts**.
- Click on the **Patient Information** and select **5-Insurance Cards**.

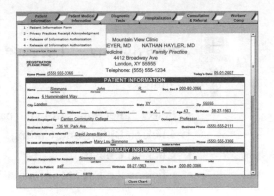

4. What is meant by PCP?

Primary Care Physician

5. What is meant by POS?

Point of Service or managed care plans that have discounts with participating physicians

6. Using the information on the insurance cards found in the medical record, what is the copay on the patient's insurance? What is the payment rate on the secondary insurance?

Copay $15.00
Secondary is   POS   80% after $500 deductible

7. Look at the back of both of the insurance cards. What do you notice when comparing the cards?

Same numbers with the exception of 1 digit in the number to call for claims

- Click **Close Chart** to return to the Billing and Coding area.
- Click the exit arrow.
- Click **Return to Map** and select **Yes** at the pop-up menu to return to the office map.

Exercise 4

Online Activity—Insurance Versus Workers' Compensation Claims

 30 minutes

- Select **Janet Jones** from the patient list.
- Click on **Billing and Coding**.
- Click on **Charts**.
- Click on the **Patient Information** tab.

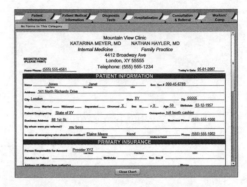

1. You will notice that in Ms. Jones' medical record, there is no information about private insurance coverage. Why is this important for this case?

2. If a patient says that he or she is injured at the workplace, or have a work-related illness, what would the medical assistant need to do before escorting the patient to the examination room? Refer to the Workers' Compensation section in Chapter 20 and Chapter 7 of the textbook if you need help locating the answer.

 • Click on the **Workers' Comp** tab.

3. What information do you find under this tab in Ms. Jones' medical record?

4. The top of the First Report of Injury states that this form is "approved as use for" two OSHA forms. What are the names of these forms?

5. If the workers' compensation carrier declares Ms. Jones' claim to be nonindustrial and refuses to pay it, is Mountain View Clinic required to write off the balance? *Use your critical thinking skills to answer this question.*

6. Can you give an example of an injury or a problem for which the insurance company might not pay if the patient had previous problems with the same or a similar diagnosis?

 • Click **Close Chart** to return to the Billing and Coding area.
   • Click the exit arrow.
   • Click **Return to Map** and select **Yes** at the pop-up menu to return to the office map.

Exercise 5

Other Activity—Proofreading and Critical Thinking Exercise

45 minutes

Jose Imero's insurance claim has been filled out by the medical assistant student. Your responsibility is to review the insurance form and make sure it is correct before billing the insurance company. There are several errors on the form. You will use the textbook, the Patient's Information Form, the Insurance Card, the Progress Notes, and the Encounter Form to ensure that everything on the form is correct. Review Chapter 21 in your textbook carefully before you begin this exercise, and use it as a tool as you review the insurance form.

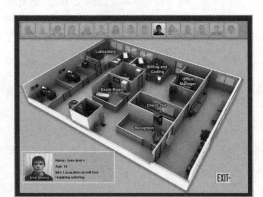

- Select **Jose Imero** from the patient list.
- Click on **Billing and Coding**.
- Click on **Charts**.
- Click on the **Patient Information** tab and select **1–Patient Information Form** to review the patient's demographic information.
- Click on the **Patient Information** tab and select **2–Insurance Cards** to verify that the insurance identification numbers are correct.
- When you get to Box 14 on the insurance claim form, click on the **Patient Medical Information** tab and select **1–Progress Notes**.
- Click **Close Chart** to return to the Billing and Coding area.
- When you get to Box 24 on the insurance claim form, click on the **Encounter Form** clipboard.
- Click **Finish** to return to the Billing and Coding area.
- Click on the **Fee Schedule** sheet to verify the insurance form has the correct amount for each service listed.
- Click **Finish** to return to the Billing and Coding area.

Important: The following instructions and notations will help as you go through the insurance form and make notations of errors.

It is indicated on Jose Imero's registration form that he is a student. For this exercise, consider his status as full-time student.

- Boxes 24 i and j should be left blank.
- For Box 25, you can locate the federal tax ID number on the Encounter Form at the top right-hand side.
- For Box 31, the office will file the claim the same date as the service was provided.
- For Box 33, the NPI number is 1234567899.

1500

HEALTH INSURANCE CLAIM FORM

APPROVED BY NATIONAL UNIFORM CLAIM COMMITTEE 08/05

☐☐ PICA   PICA ☐☐

1. MEDICARE ☐ (Medicare #)	MEDICAID ☐ (Medicaid #)	TRICARE CHAMPUS ☐ (Sponsor's SSN)	CHAMPVA ☐ (Member ID#)	GROUP HEALTH PLAN ☒ (SSN or ID)	FECA BLK LUNG ☐ (SSN)	OTHER ☐ (ID)	1a. INSURED'S I.D. NUMBER (For Program in Item 1)

1a. INSURED'S I.D. NUMBER — YAM 150221114

2. PATIENT'S NAME (Last Name, First Name, Middle Initial)
Imero, Jose

3. PATIENT'S BIRTH DATE — MM 03 DD 15 YY 91   SEX M ☒ F ☐

4. INSURED'S NAME (Last Name, First Name, Middle Initial)
IMERO ANTONIO

5. PATIENT'S ADDRESS (No., Street)
253 Lindhurst Way

6. PATIENT RELATIONSHIP TO INSURED
Self ☐ Spouse ☐ Child ☒ Other ☐

7. INSURED'S ADDRESS (No., Street)
4628 Mission Way

CITY **London**   STATE **XY**

8. PATIENT STATUS
Single ☐ Married ☐ Other ☐

CITY **Trumball**   STATE **YZ**

ZIP CODE **55555**   TELEPHONE (Include Area Code) **(555) 555-5455**

Employed ☐ Full-Time Student ☐ Part-Time Student ☒

ZIP CODE **99999**   TELEPHONE (Include Area Code) **(555) 555-7878**

9. OTHER INSURED'S NAME (Last Name, First Name, Middle Initial)

10. IS PATIENT'S CONDITION RELATED TO:

11. INSURED'S POLICY GROUP OR FECA NUMBER
1822

a. OTHER INSURED'S POLICY OR GROUP NUMBER

a. EMPLOYMENT? (Current or Previous) YES ☐ NO ☒

a. INSURED'S DATE OF BIRTH — MM 12 DD 12 YY 74   SEX M ☒ F ☐

b. OTHER INSURED'S DATE OF BIRTH MM DD YY   SEX M ☐ F ☐

b. AUTO ACCIDENT? YES ☐ NO ☒   PLACE (State)

b. EMPLOYER'S NAME OR SCHOOL NAME
Sunshine Foods

c. EMPLOYER'S NAME OR SCHOOL NAME

c. OTHER ACCIDENT? YES ☒ NO ☐

c. INSURANCE PLAN NAME OR PROGRAM NAME
Blue Cross/Blue Shield

d. INSURANCE PLAN NAME OR PROGRAM NAME

10d. RESERVED FOR LOCAL USE

d. IS THERE ANOTHER HEALTH BENEFIT PLAN?
YES ☐ NO ☒   If yes, return to and complete item 9 a-d.

READ BACK OF FORM BEFORE COMPLETING & SIGNING THIS FORM.
12. PATIENT'S OR AUTHORIZED PERSON'S SIGNATURE I authorize the release of any medical or other information necessary to process this claim. I also request payment of government benefits either to myself or to the party who accepts assignment below.

SIGNED **Signature on File**   DATE

13. INSURED'S OR AUTHORIZED PERSON'S SIGNATURE I authorize payment of medical benefits to the undersigned physician or supplier for services described below.

SIGNED **Signature on File**

14. DATE OF CURRENT: MM 05 DD 01 YY 07   ILLNESS (First symptom) OR INJURY (Accident) OR PREGNANCY(LMP)

15. IF PATIENT HAS HAD SAME OR SIMILAR ILLNESS. GIVE FIRST DATE MM DD YY

16. DATES PATIENT UNABLE TO WORK IN CURRENT OCCUPATION
FROM MM DD YY   TO MM DD YY

17. NAME OF REFERRING PROVIDER OR OTHER SOURCE

17a.
17b. NPI

18. HOSPITALIZATION DATES RELATED TO CURRENT SERVICES
FROM MM DD YY   TO MM DD YY

19. RESERVED FOR LOCAL USE

20. OUTSIDE LAB? YES ☐ NO ☒ $ CHARGES

21. DIAGNOSIS OR NATURE OF ILLNESS OR INJURY (Relate Items 1, 2, 3 or 4 to Item 24E by Line)

1. Open Wound L foot 8 cm w/ complications   3.
2.   4.

22. MEDICAID RESUBMISSION CODE   ORIGINAL REF. NO.

23. PRIOR AUTHORIZATION NUMBER

24. A. DATE(S) OF SERVICE From MM DD YY	To MM DD YY	B. PLACE OF SERVICE	C. EMG	D. PROCEDURES, SERVICES, OR SUPPLIES (Explain Unusual Circumstances) CPT/HCPCS MODIFIER	E. DIAGNOSIS POINTER	F. $ CHARGES	G. DAYS OR UNITS	H. EPSDT Family Plan	I. ID. QUAL	J. RENDERING PROVIDER ID. #
1	05 05 07	05 01 07	11		Est. visit, Level II	laceration	45 00	1	N	NPI	
2					Tetanus	laceration	15 00	1	N	NPI	
3					Immun. Single	laceration	25 00	1	N	NPI	
4					Surgical Tray	laceration	15 00	1	N	NPI	
5					Wound Repair	laceration	175 00	1	N	NPI	
6										NPI	

25. FEDERAL TAX I.D. NUMBER   SSN EIN
123456789 ☐☐

26. PATIENT'S ACCOUNT NO.

27. ACCEPT ASSIGNMENT? (For govt. claims, see back) YES ☒ NO ☐

28. TOTAL CHARGE $ **275 00**

29. AMOUNT PAID $ **25 00**

30. BALANCE DUE $ **250 00**

31. SIGNATURE OF PHYSICIAN OR SUPPLIER INCLUDING DEGREES OR CREDENTIALS (I certify that the statements on the reverse apply to this bill and are made a part thereof.)
SOF
SIGNED   05012007 DATE

32. SERVICE FACILITY LOCATION INFORMATION
44 BROADWAY
LONDON, XY, 55555
a. NPI   b.

33. BILLING PROVIDER INFO & PH # ( )
NATHAN HAYLER MD
4412 BROADWAY
LONDON, XY, 55555
a. **1234567899** b.

NUCC Instruction Manual available at: www.nucc.org   APPROVED OMB-0938-0999 FORM CMS-1500 (08/05)

1. Below, list any errors you found as you reviewed Jose Imero's insurance claim form.

- Click the exit arrow.
- Click **Return to Map**, then click **Yes** at the pop-up menu to return to the office map or click Exit the Program.

Bookkeeping

Patients: All

Learning Objectives:

- Post daily entries on the day sheet and prepare bank deposits at the end of the day.
- Process credit balances, NSF checks, and checks from collection agencies.
- Process credit balances and complete necessary steps to process a refund, including preparation of a check.
- Reconcile a bank statement.
- Maintain a petty cash fund.
- Discuss the maintenance of records for accounting and banking purposes.
- Discuss the importance of managing accounts payable promptly.

Overview:

In this lesson the basic bookkeeping procedures will be accomplished. All patients will be added to the day sheet, along with the payments and the NSF check received in today's mail. A deposit record will be prepared. The steps for reconciliation of the bank statement and maintenance of records for accounting purposes will also be covered.

Exercise 1

Online Activity—Posting Charges to Ledger Cards

30 minutes

- Sign in to Mountain View Clinic.
- Select **Jade Wong** from the patient list.
- Click on **Billing and Coding**.
- Click on the **Encounter Form** clipboard and **Fee Schedule** sheet as needed to complete the following questions.

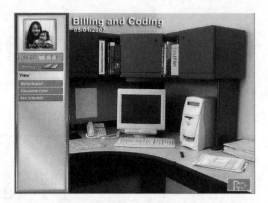

1. a. Using the Encounter Form for Jade Wong, begin completing the blank ledger card below.
   b. In the column marked Professional Service, list each individual service provided, but do not enter any fee or balance information.
   c. After the last service has been entered, be sure to record that the co-pay was collected and enter the amount in the Payment column.
   d. Fill in the fees charged for the listed services and calculate the balances.

   Important: The balance should be corrected line by line as each service or payment is added or subtracted.

Mountain View Clinic
Patient Ledger

Patient Name:

Insurance Type:

Date	Professional Service	Fee ($)	Payment ($)	Adj. ($)	Prev. Bal. ($)	New Balance ($)
Totals:						

2. After filling in the services, fees, and payments for Jade's current visit, should the ledger card be totaled as indicated at the bottom of the card? Refer to the textbook, if needed, and explain your answer.

3. How did the medical assistant know what Jade's copay was?

 • Click **Finish** to return to the Billing and Coding area.

• Click the exit arrow.

• Click **Return to Map** and select **Yes** at the pop-up menu to return to the office map.

Exercise 2

 Online Activity—Posting Entries to a Day Sheet

 60 minutes

1. In this activity you will post charges and payments for the patients who were seen in the office today, using the day sheet on the next page. Note that the distribution column indicates which physician, Dr. Hayler or Dr. Meyer, provided care to the patient. The amount of money the patient paid should be written in one of those columns in addition to the payment column.

a. In the Patient Name column on the blank day sheet below, list the patients in the following order: Jade Wong, Louise Parlet, Hu Huang, Rhea Davison, Jesus Santo, Jean Deere, Tristan Tsosie, Wilson Metcalf, Renee Anderson, Jose Imero, Shaunti Begay, Janet Jones, Kevin McKinzie, John R. Simmons, and Teresa Hernandez.

b. Select **Jade Wong** from the patient list. Then click on **Check Out** on the office map. Once in the Check Out area, click on the **Encounter Form** clipboard.

c. Using one line per patient, complete each column on the day sheet using the Total Charges, Previous Balance, and Amount Received information listed on the Encounter Form. Refer back to the ledger card in Exercise 1 to confirm your totals. (Note: Unlike the ledger card, the Professional Service column on the day sheet is a summary description of the visit.)

d. For the purposes of this exercise, also make a note next to each patient's name to indicate whether the patient paid by cash, check, or credit card. If payment was made by check, include the check number.

e. Click **Finish** to close the Encounter Form. Click the exit arrow, then click **Return to Map** and select **Yes** at the pop-up menu to return to the office map and select the next patient.

Repeat the above steps by selecting each patient and opening his or her Encounter Form at Check Out.

f. When you finish recording the information for the last patient on the list, remain at the office map to continue with the next question.

Mountain View Clinic
Daysheet

Date	Professional Service	Fee	Payment	Adjustment	New Balance	Old Balance	Patient's Name	Distribution	
								Dr. Hayler	Dr. Meyer
TOTALS									**TOTALS**

- Click on **Reception**.
- Click on the **Stackable Trays**.
- Click the numbers or arrows at the top of the page to examine and read each piece of mail.

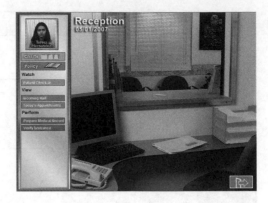

2. a. On the blank day sheet on the next page, record any payments received by the clinic and any charges paid by the clinic in the appropriate columns.

   b. Be sure to include a description of the payment/charge and the patient's name.

   c. For the purposes of this exercise, make a note of the bank and check number next to the name of any patient who paid by check.

   d. To complete the remaining columns, click **Finish** to return to the Reception area.

   e. Click the exit arrow, then click **Return to Map** and select **Yes** at the pop-up menu to return to the office map

   f. Click on **Office Manager** and then on the **Day Sheet** document to find any previous balance information. Recalculate the balance and record in the New Balance column.

   g. Mark Bonsel's previous account balance was zero ("0") before you received the NSF check. The NSF check shows that it was paid on April 7, 2007, but it does not indicate what it was for, other than a balance. Assume it was for a Level II New Patient Visit, which would be $65.00 on the date of April 7, 2007.

   h. *Note:* A copy of Sarah Anita's EOB from Blue Cross/Blue Shield was received in the mail. The insurance payment and adjustment were already posted on the day sheet and her ledger in the office manager's section of the Office. The copy of the EOB in the mail will not need posting again.

   i. Recalculate the balance and record it in the New Balance column.

Mountain View Clinic
Daysheet

Date	Professional Service	Fee	Payment	Adjustment	New Balance	Old Balance	Patient's Name	Distribution Dr. Hayler	Distribution Dr. Meyer

TOTALS

TOTALS

• Click **Finish** to return to the manager's office.
• Remain in the Office Manager area to continue to Exercise 4.

Exercise 3

 Writing Activity—Preparing a Bank Deposit

 15 minutes

Using the information recorded in the completed day sheets in Exercise 2, you will now prepare a bank deposit (both front and back) for the accounts receivable for the day. Be sure the total on the deposit slip balances with the total of receivables on the day sheet.

1. Below, complete the front side of the deposit slip.

DEPOSIT SLIP

Clarion National Bank
90 Grape Vine Road
London, XY 55555-0001

Mountain View Clinic
4412 Broadway
London, XY 55555

Date: _____

CASH			TOTAL
	Currency	$_____	
	Coin	$_____	$_____
	Total Cash		$_____
CHECKS	See other side for detail		$_____
- CASH REC'D			$_____
NET DEPOSIT			$_____

_____
SIGN HERE IN TELLER'S PRESENCE FOR CASH RECEIVED

2. Below, complete the back portion of the bank deposit slip. (*Note:* The bank number cannot be obtained from the day sheet. For the purposes of this exercise, use the check number as a substitute.)

BANK DEPOSIT DETAIL

PAYMENTS

BANK NUMBER	BY CHECK OR PMO	BY COIN OR CURRENCY	CREDIT CARD	
TOTALS				
CURRENCY				
COIN				
CHECKS				
CREDIT CARDS				
TOTAL RECEIPTS				
LESS CREDIT CARD $				
TOTAL DEPOSIT				
DEPOSIT DATE _____				

Exercise 4

Online Activity—Processing Credit Balances

20 minutes

- Click on **Day Sheet** document.

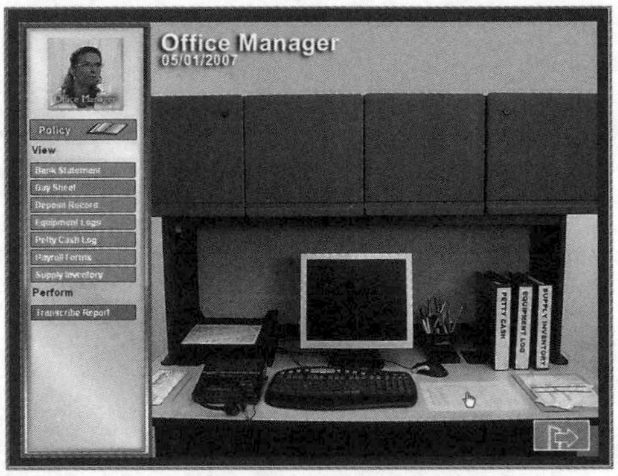

1. Two patients listed on the day sheet have overpaid, which resulted in a credit balance denoted by a parenthesis around the amount that was overpaid. Betsy Dunworthy overpaid by $20.00 and her refund was already processed. What is the name of the other patient who should receive a refund, and how much money should he receive?

2. Using the blank check below, process the outstanding refund for payment.

173975

DATE:	
TO:	
FOR:	
ACCOUNT No.	
AMOUNT PAID	$

MOUNTAIN VIEW CLINIC
4412 Broadway
London, XY 55555

173975

94-72/1224

Date: ______________________

Pay to the order of: ______________________

______________________ *Dollars* $

Clarion National Bank
Member FDIC
90 Grape Vine Road
London, XY 55555-0001

____
Authorized Signature

⑈005503⑈ 446782011⑈ 678800470

- Click **Finish** to return to the manager's office.

Exercise 5

Online Activity—Maintaining Petty Cash Fund

30 minutes

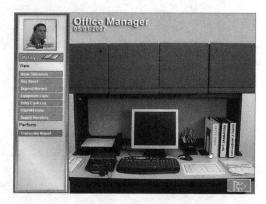

- Click on the **Petty Cash Binder**.

1. Petty cash was used to pay for the mailing of a certified letter. What is the receipt number and date from this transaction?

2. On 5/1/07, the administrative medical assistant was asked to obtain soft drinks for an office celebration to be held that afternoon. These were bought at Sav-A-Grocery for the amount of $24.56. She also mailed a large package at the post office. The cost for mailing the package was $15.08. Using the form below, fill out the first petty cash voucher.

Date: _____   Nu.. _____

PETTY CASH VOUCHER

For: _____

Charge to: _____

_____

Approved by: Received by:

_____   _____

Authorized Signature

3. Now fill out the second petty cash voucher.

Date: _____   No.: _____

PETTY CASH VOUCHER

For: _____

Charge to: _____

_____

Approved by: _____   Received by: _____

_____   _____

Authorized Signature

4. Using the completed petty cash vouchers from questions 2 and 3, update the petty cash log below accordingly. Be sure to distribute the expenses to the proper expense column.

NO.	DATE	DESCRIPTION	AMOUNT	OFFICE EXP.	AUTO.	MISC.	BALANCE
	2/16/2007	Fund Established (check #217)					200.00
101	2/24/2007	Certified Letter	3.74	3.74			196.26
102	3/1/2007	Staff Meeting/Lunch	24.60			24.60	171.66
103	3/6/2007	Coffee	4.32			4.32	167.34
104	3/8/2007	Tympanic Thermometer	38.00	38.00			129.34
105	3/8/2007	Parking Fee	6.00		6.00		123.34
106	4/1/2007	Staff Meeting/Lunch	27.43			27.43	95.91
107	4/13/2007	Miscellaneous Supplies	9.01	9.01			86.90
108	4/21/2007	Patient Birthday Cards	12.17	12.17			74.73

5. Office policy states that petty cash should be replenished when the amount falls below $50. Use the blank check below to replenish the petty cash fund to the full $200 balance as required by the office policy. Then, using the updated petty cash log in question 4, verify the petty cash fund balances by totaling all the columns, and add this transaction to the log.

173976

DATE:	
TO:	
FOR:	
ACCOUNT NO.	
AMOUNT PAID	$

MOUNTAIN VIEW CLINIC
4412 Broadway
London, XY 55555   173976

                                           94-72/1224

Date: _____

Pay to the order of: _____

_____ Dollars $ _____

Clarion National Bank
        Member FDIC
90 Grape Vine Road
London, XY 55555-0001   _____
                                     Authorized Signature

II 005503 II 4467882011 II 678800470

- Click **Finish** to return to the manager's office.
- Click the exit arrow.
- Click **Return to Map** and select **Yes** at the pop-up menu to return to the office map.
- Select **Jose Imero** from the patient list.
- Click on **Check Out**.
- Under the Watch heading, click on Patient Check-Out and watch the video.

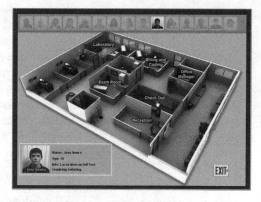

6. What are the ethical implications of Kristin asking another medical assistant for money from petty cash?

- Click the **X** on the video screen to close the video.
- Click the exit arrow.
- Click **Return to Map** and select **Yes** at the pop-up menu to return to the office map.

Exercise 6

Online Activity—Managing Accounts Payable

30 minutes

- Click on **Reception**.
- Click on the **Stackable Trays**.
- Click the numbers or arrows at the top of the page to examine and read pieces 8 and 9.

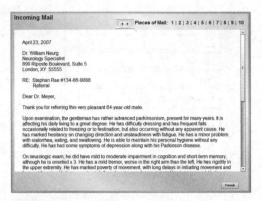

1. Indicate whether each of the following statements is true or false.

a. _____ When accounts payable arrive, the date for payment with discounts should be noted.

b. _____ It really does not matter what day of the month an accounts payable payment is made, as long as it is paid before the next billing cycle.

c. _____ Invoices should be marked with the date and check number, as well as the initials of the person preparing the check.

d. _____ All accounts payables should be checked against invoices and packing slips before payment is made.

e. _____ All vendors will present invoices before payment is due.

2. What information does the accounts payable person need to correctly process and post the payment of the invoices (pieces 8 and 9 of the incoming mail)? Select all that apply.

_____ Invoice number

_____ Company name

_____ Name of the customer service representative

_____ Date of check

_____ Account number

_____ Company address

_____ Company phone number

_____ Name of the company's bank

_____ Company's bank account number

_____ Type of expense

_____ Amount of the check

_____ Invoice date

_____ Check number

- Click **Finish** to return to the Reception area.
- Click the exit arrow.
- Click **Return to Map** and select **Yes** at the pop-up menu to return to the office map.

Exercise 7

 ## Online Activity—Reconciling a Bank Statement

 30 minutes

The clinic's bank statement arrives in today's mail. This is found in the manager's office. She is extremely busy and asks that you take the time to reconcile the statement for her.

- Click on **Office Manager**.
- Click on the **Bank Statement** file folder.

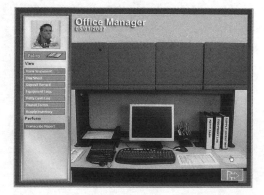

1. a. Using the check ledger below, review the bank statement and check off each deposit, check, withdrawal, ATM transaction, or credit listed on the statement.

   b. If the statement shows any interest paid to the account, any service charges, bank fees, automatic payments, or ATM transactions withdrawn from the account that are not listed on the check ledger, make an entry for those items now and recalculate the account balance in the ledger.

No.	Date	Description	Payment/ Debit	Ref	Deposit/ Credit	Balance
1216	3/5/2007	Rocke Medical	$625.00			$9,264.35
1217	3/5/2007	Wal Store	$38.46			$9,225.89
1218	3/6/2007	Lorenz Equipment	$1,006.00			$8,219.89
1219	3/8/2007	Office Station	$199.43			$8,020.46
	3/10/2007	Dep. Daily Trans			$1,050.00	$10,833.46
1220	3/10/2007	West Electric	$93.99			$7,926.47
	3/12/2007	Dep. Daily Trans			$2,008.00	$9,934.47
1221	3/12/2007	Office Depot	$102.01			$9,832.46
1222	3/12/2007	Video Inc.	$49.00			$9,783.46
	3/15/2007	Dep. Daily Trans			$1,002.00	$11,835.46
1223	3/17/2007	Bonus	$200.00			$12,560.46
1224	3/17/2007	Bonus	$200.00			$12,360.46
1225	3/17/2007	Bonus	$200.00			$12,160.46
	3/20/2007	Dep. Daily Trans			$925.00	$12,760.46
1226	3/21/2007	Jamison Medical	$2,024.20			$10,136.26
1227	3/22/2007	Healthy Living Magazine	$32.95			$10,103.31
1228	3/22/2007	Greater London Electric	$422.00			$9,681.31
1229	3/24/2007	Office Station	$344.70			$9,336.61
1230	3/25/2007	Summer Oxygen	$230.99			$9,105.62
	3/27/2007	Dep. Daily Trans			$1,550.00	$10,655.62

2. Now complete the bank reconciliation worksheet below.

THIS WORKSHEET IS PROVIDED TO HELP YOU BALANCE YOUR ACCOUNT

1. Go through your register and mark each check, withdrawal, Express ATM transaction, payment, deposit or other credit listed on your statement. Be sure that your register shows any interest paid into your account, and any service charges, bank fees, automatic payments, or Express Transfers withdrawn from your account during this statement period.

2. Using the chart below, list any outstanding checks, Express ATM withdrawals, payments or any other withdrawals (including any from previous months) that are listed in your register but are not shown on this statement.

3. Balance your account by filling in the spaces below.

ITEMS OUTSTANDING		
NUMBER	**AMOUNT**	
TOTAL		

ENTER

The ENDING BALANCE shown on this statement -------------------------------- $ _____ __

ADD

Any deposits listed in your register or $ _____ __
transfers into your account which are $ _____ __
not shown on this statement $ _____ __
                                                +$ _____ __

TOTAL --- +$ _____ __

CALCULATE THE SUBTOTAL --- $ _____ __

SUBTRACT

The total outstanding checks and
Withdrawals from the chart at the left -------------------------------------- $ _____ __

CALCULATE THE ENDING BALANCE

This amount should be the same as
The current balance shown in your
Check register -- $ _____ __

- Click **Finish** to return to the manager's office.
- Click the exit arrow.
- Click **Return to Map** and select **Yes** at the pop-up menu to return to the office map or click **Exit the Program**.

Payroll Procedures

Reading Assignment: Chapter 24—Management of Practice Finances
• Payroll Records

Patients: None

Learning Objectives:

• Process the employee payroll.
• Locate federal tax withholding resources by using the Internet

Overview:

For administrative medical assistants, the task of preparing an employee payroll may be a routine function. This lesson will give you practice in preparing payroll for employees.

Exercise 1

Online Activity—Processing Payroll

 20 minutes

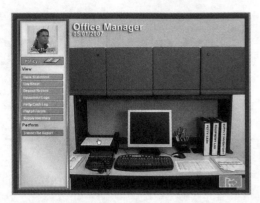

- Sign in to Mountain View Clinic.
- Click on **Office Manager**.
- Click on the **Stackable Trays**.
- The time sheet for employee Cathy Wright will appear first. Review and confirm that the number of hours have been calculated correctly.
- Next, click on the down arrow next to Person and select **Susan Bronski**.
- Review Susan Bronski's and confirm that the number of hours have been calculated correctly.

1. Cathy Wright's total number of hours worked: _____

   Susan Bronski's total number of hours worked: _____

2. Cathy Wright has been employed by the clinic for 10 years. Her salary is $18.00 per hour for the first 80 hours and $27.00 per hour for any hours over 80 during the 2-week pay period. Compute the gross pay for Cathy for the 2-week period.

3. Susan Bronski is a relatively new employee who is making $15.00 per hour for the first 80 hours and $20 per hour for hours over 80. Complete the gross pay for Susan for the 2-week period.

- Now review the W-4 form filled out by each employee.
- To view Cathy Wright's W-4 form, first make sure her name is selected from the drop-down menu next to Person. Next, click on the down arrow next to Form and select W-4. Review her form.
- To view Susan Bronski's W-4 form, select her name from the drop-down menu next to Person.

4. Cathy Wright elected to have her federal taxes withheld under which designation?

_____ Single

_____ Married

_____ Married, but withhold at the higher single rate

5. The number of allowances claimed by Cathy Wright is _____.

6. Did Cathy Wright elect to have any additional money withheld from her paycheck for federal taxes? If yes, how much?

7. Susan Bronski will have her federal taxes withheld under which designation?

_____ Single

_____ Married

_____ Married, but withhold at the higher single rate

8. The number of allowances claimed by Susan Bronski is _____.

9. Did Susan Bronski elect to have any additional money withheld from her paycheck for federal taxes? If yes, how much?

Exercise 2

Writing Activity—Calculating Net Pay

30 minutes

The IRS updates the federal tax tables each year. The tables we are using for this activity are 2010 tables for Single and Married Persons BiWeekly Payroll (you will choose which table to use based on the employee's filing status). Go to the Evolve course website. Click on Course Documents to view the 2010 tax tables. If you are instructed by your teacher to obtain the most recent copy of the schedules, go to the IRS website at www.irs.gov. Each state may have its own amount for the state withholding, but for this exercise we will use 1%.

1. Calculate the total withholding allowance for Cathy Wright and Susan Bronski.

   Total withholding allowance for Cathy Wright: _____

   Total withholding allowance for Susan Bronski: _____

2. Now subtract the total withholding allowance from each employee's gross pay to calculate the adjusted gross pay.

   Cathy Wright's adjusted gross pay: _____

   Susan Bronski's adjusted gross pay: _____

3. Account for the following additional deductions for Cathy Wright: Medicare = 1.45%, Social Security = 6.2%, Health Insurance = $125 per pay period, State Income Tax = 1%, Retirement Plan = $150 per pay period.

Federal Income Tax	
Medicare	
Social Security	
Health Insurance	
State Income Tax	
Retirement Plan	

4. What is the net pay for Cathy Wright?

5. a. Using the correct tax table, calculate the correct deductions for Susan Bronski, who will file as head of household.
   b. Account for the following additional deductions for Susan Bronski: Medicare = 1.45%, Social Security = 6.2%, Health Insurance = $175 per pay period, State Income Tax = 1%, Savings Plan = $50 per pay period, Additional Tax Withholding from W-4 = $190.00.

Federal Income Tax	
Medicare	
Social Security	
Health Insurance	
State Income Tax	
Savings Deduction	
Additional Tax Withholding	

6. What is the net pay for Susan Bronski?

Exercise 3

 Online Activity—Writing the Check for Payroll

 15 minutes

You are now ready to prepare and issue the payroll checks for Cathy Wright and Susan Bronski. To obtain the correct ending date for the pay period, return to the employees' time sheets by clicking on Payroll Forms in the manager's office. Date the checks for the Monday following the end of the pay period.

1. Prepare Cathy Wright's payroll check below.

PERIOD ENDING	EARNINGS			DEDUCTIONS									NET PAY	
HOURS WORKED REG. OT	REGULAR	OVERTIME	TOTAL	FEDERAL INCOME TAX	FICA TAX	STATE INCOME TAX	SDI TAX	HEALTH INS.	SAVINGS	MEDICARE	MISC DED.	TOTAL DED.	AMOUNT

CHECK # 173977   **Employee:**

MOUNTAIN VIEW CLINIC   173977
4412 Broadway
London, XY 55555   94-72/1224

                                         Date: _____

Pay to the order of: _____

_____ *Dollars* $ [   ]

Clarion National Bank
          Member FDIC
90 Grape Vine Road   _____
London, XY 55555-0001
                                                    Authorized Signature

⑊ 005503 ⑊ 446782011 ⑊ 678800470

2. Prepare Susan Bronski's payroll check below.

PERIOD ENDING	EARNINGS			DEDUCTIONS								NET PAY	
HOURS WORKED REG. OT	REGULAR	OVERTIME	TOTAL	FEDERAL INCOME TAX	FICA TAX	STATE INCOME TAX	SDI TAX	HEALTH INS.	SAVINGS	MEDICARE	MISC DED.	TOTAL DED.	AMOUNT

CHECK # 173978   **Employee:**

MOUNTAIN VIEW CLINIC   173978
4412 Broadway
London, XY 55555   94-72/1.224
                                                  Date: _____

Pay to the order of: _____

_____ Dollars $ [   ]

Clarion National Bank
        Member FDIC
90 Grape Vine Road   _____
London, XY 55555-0001   *Authorized Signature*

|| 005503 || 46782011 || 678800470